After
a
Fall

This book is dedicated with love and gratitude to
Ernest Lockridge

After a Fall

A Sociomedical Sojourn

&

LAUREL RICHARDSON

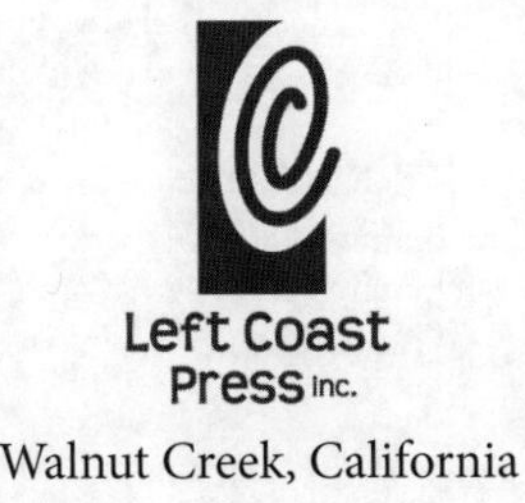

Left Coast
Press Inc.

Walnut Creek, California

ISBN 978-1-61132-316-0 hardcover
ISBN 978-1-61132-317-7 paperback
ISBN 978-1-61132-318-4 institutional eBook
ISBN 978-1-61132-715-1 consumer eBook

Library of Congress Cataloging-in-Publication Data
Richardson, Laurel.
  After a fall : a sociomedical sojourn / Laurel Richardson.
     p. ;   cm.
  Includes bibliographical references.
    ISBN 978-1-61132-316-0 (hardback : alk. paper) — ISBN 978-1-61132-317-7 (pbk. : alk. paper) — ISBN 978-1-61132-318-4 (institutional ebook) — ISBN 978-1-61132-715-1 (consumer ebook)
   I. Title.
   [DNLM: 1. Patients—Personal Narratives. 2. Foot Injuries—Personal Narratives. 3. Skilled Nursing Facilities. WE 880]
    362.16—dc23   2012050070

Printed in the United States of America

The paper used in this publication meets the minimum requirements of American National Standard for Information Sciences—Permanence of Paper for Printed Library Materials, ANSI/NISO Z39.48–1992.

Design and production: Detta Penna

Cover image: Outside the Bellemont by Ernest Lockeridge, 2013.

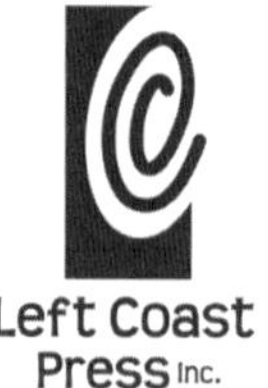

LEFT COAST PRESS, INC.
1630 North Main Street, #400
Walnut Creek, CA 94596
http://www.LCoastPress.com

Contents

Come, butterfly
It's late—
We've miles to go together.

BASHŌ

CHAPTER 1

Fear of Falling

January 5

I have frequently driven past the Bellemont, but now I am in it. An ambulance brought me here on a gurney. Two orderlies carried me in and Ernest carried my suitcase in and unpacked it. It is late afternoon. There are no fetid smells. My left foot and calf are swaddled in six feet of Ace bandage. The nerve block has not worn off, a DonJoy IceMan chills my ankle, and Vicodin circulates in my bloodstream. There is no pain.

Funny to write those four words—"there is no pain"—without my customary introduction: God is Love. I will do it now: *God is Love, there is no pain.* My Christian Science-inclined father taught me this mantra when I was six and had broken my arm falling on the ice because I tried skating like the boys, with my hands cupped together behind my back. I trudged through the rest of that Chicago winter with my left arm slung in a piece of torn sheet Father had tied around my neck, the bone healing itself, the bone mending crooked, my first grade teacher the only adult noticing, telling my mother to bring me to a doctor. She did so without my father's consent. Looking at my plaster cast, Father shook his head in anger and disappointment. Ever since then I have associated being incapacitated or sick with the neglect, disapproval, and anger of those who are supposed to love and protect me.

It is as if I am living in a long-term awful story, a plot that says if I am ill it is because I have been "bad"; and if I am "bad," I deserve "punishment." Maybe that's why I have such a high pain tolerance. Maybe that's why I never took an aspirin, never registered a headache, until after my first day of teaching. Maybe that's why I chose to deliver both of my sons through natural childbirth, and still contend that "there was no pain," only labor. Maybe that's why so many other things rankle around in me, unresolved: to acknowledge them is to acknowledge pain.

My private room in the Bellemont looks out on an enclosed courtyard with picnic benches, sensible chairs, and a roofed-over smoking lounge. I am lying in bed in my hospital gown in the Rehabilitation Wing, Hallway 100, Room 112. It is good to know where I am. In my room are a clothes closet, bed-table, large round table, four wooden chairs, two comfy chairs, a wall clock, and a bulletin board to which a blue snowflake January calendar has been pinned. There is no mirror.

Looking out my window, I see a church steeple, and a surprisingly blue sky for Ohio in January. For the next two weeks, I am not allowed to put any weight on my left foot. That is okay. I feel at home here.

"I'll go home and eat some dinner," Ernest says. "I'll get the Papillons and come back." He kisses me.

CHECK HALL 100 EXIT CHECK HALL 100 EXIT CHECK HALL 100 EXIT RRRRRRRRIIIIIINNNNNNGGGGGG RRRRRRRRIIIIIINNNNNNGGGGGG

A robotic school-marmish voice scolds us over the public address system. One of the Bellemont's wings is for dementia patients, so I think codes have to be entered before opening the outside doors, but I don't know that for sure because no one from the facility has been here to see me yet. I think Ernest set off the alarm.

I had put off my ankle surgery. It was irrational, I know, but I feared I would die—or worse. I had become obsessed with getting my affairs in order: I had new legal documents drawn up; I finished everything on my academic plate; I sent "thinking of you" notes and emails to friends; I paid all my bills, settled all accounts; I spent special time with my sons; I got a year's grooming appointments for my Papillon dogs, Bashi and Lily—and, for good measure ordered a paving-stone in their names for WOOF, the new Worthington Off-Leash Dog-Park; I showed Ernest where I kept all my important documents. I threw out my old panties.

I am not dead, but I am sleepy.

"Hi, I'm Jamal." A young African-American man enters my room. "Sorry, I'm late. I'm your nurse's aide until eleven p.m." He checks his Swatch and adjusts his tortoise-shell glasses. His biceps flex.

Jamal asks permission to go through my belongings so he can count and register them. He looks uncomfortable touching my clothing.

"Oh, just write something down," I say. "I didn't bring anything of value."

"Your laptop," he says. "I'd better put that in your dresser. Your iPad, too. Things can get stolen." He takes my vitals, refills my DonJon IceMan with ice, shows me how the push-buttons on my bed work, and helps me to use the bedside commode. Both of us are embarrassed.

"Have you worked here long?" I ask.

"Just started. You're my first patient."

I hear the familiar jingle-jangle of dog tags coming down the hallway.

"Ernest, meet Jamal," I say, as Ernest puts Bashi and Lily on the bed with me.

"What kind of dogs are they?" Jamal asks. He looks apprehensive.

"They're sweethearts," Ernest says. "Papillons."

"French for butterfly," Jamal says, gingerly touching their ears.

Lily sniffs my wrapped-up foot. Bashi gives me dog-kisses.

"Dog-nap," Ernest says, and the dogs and I settle down on my hospital bed. Ernest settles down with his Kindle, a gift for his seventy-third birthday from our Columbus "blended family." Like so many other "blended" families that arise out of divorces, ours is not a purée. We have chunks that collide, edges that have not worn down. Ernest cried when he read the card signed by all ten of us.

Ah! The blended-family? I smile at how the nineteenth-century metaphor of the "melting pot," a harmonious society in which new immigrants embrace a common culture, has been transformed into a "blender" and applied to contemporary family life, where presumably, and desirably, the adults and children will live in unanimity. But just as melting is a questionable and non-attainable ideal for American society, so, I think, blending is for step-families. *Salad, anyone?*

"Please close the door when you leave," I say to Jamal. He does. The hallway noise is blessedly quieted.

"Rest well, Darling," Ernest says, whispering my favorite endearment. "Time for me to go, too." He kisses me, collects the dogs, and off he and the dogs go into the night. I feel safe.

"We're leaving for Hawaii tomorrow," Bev says, "so we wanted to see you tonight." Bev is in my memoir-writing group—seven women who have been meeting bi-monthly for twelve years. Bev is always well turned-out. Tonight she is wearing a black skirt-suit, knee-high black boots and a cape of many colors

"You're looking good," her husband Craig says, as he gives me a tentative hug. His left shoulder droops from post-polio syndrome. Craig has been jostling with retirement from his university professorship. It is hard to let go of the identity, status, and perks that being a professor confer. You pass as smart, even if you aren't; you can claim to know more than you do, and others accept the sham. You set the rhythm of your days, and can demand everyone *be quiet and shut-up* because you are working on your seminal project.

But when you retire, you become dispensable. When I asked for post-retirement office space, my startled department chair said, "Why, I thought Emeriti just crawled into the woodwork." When Ernest updated his *Who's Who* entry to reflect his retirement from the English Department, his entry was dropped. Career consultants say that many professors feel lost after retiring because so much of their lives have been tied up in the university. Their work, their friends, and even their vacations—often tied to their disciplines' scholarly meetings—are integrated. Some care deeply that they won't be passing on the knowledge they have accumulated. Many faculty have built programs, labs, and specialties that they fear will be demolished when they retire because their university will likely replace them with adjuncts rather than tenure-track faculty. The adjuncts are neither hired for, nor committed to, stewarding the existing programs.

Larger issues bear down on the faculty, too. Economic uncertainty has created "portfolio phobia." What faculty could once count upon—their pensions or investments—now seem fragile and under assault. Universities have not rushed in with economic incentives (such as buy-outs, phase-outs, or deferred annuities) to ease the faculty's financial fears. And then there are the health-care issues. With no mandatory retirement, and no mandatory replacement with tenure-track profes-sors, and with a plethora of emotional, social, and economic concerns, it is not surprising that faculty commonly put off retiring until they fear that they "might fall off the stage."

I empathize with Craig's difficulty in letting go. I'm still working on accepting being retired, on accepting my title, Emeritus Professor of Sociology. It's been nearly a decade since I taught my last univer-sity class. But I am *not* retired: I write, I give workshops, I serve on journals, and I mentor. But mostly I work *pro bono*. I don't get paid. Making money for one's labor is the hallmark of *societal* value. So, I—and other Emeriti faculty who do as I do—have left not only the pres-tige that came with being a university professor, we have given up our status as employed earners. Yet, there is comfort in not being judged by the size of my salary.

"For so many years, Craig," I say, "I avoided uttering the word *retired* ... almost like how forty years ago people avoided uttering the word *cancer*."

"Retirement has all these negative connotations." Craig shakes his head. "Like worn out. Tired. Outdated. Broken. Useless. And that's not how I like to think of myself."

"Nor should we," I say.

"Most retirees today are pretty fit," Bev says in her upbeat Mem-phis accent.

"And that's why pop culture has come up with a slew of new names for retirement," I say. "Rewire, re-tire, advanced, sage-age, and –my fa-vorite –jubilated. Like we've been lifted into a paradise."

"Not very catchy," Bev says.

"And none has won the re-naming game," I add.

Snort. Gasp. Snort. Gag. Loud guttural sounds echo through the corridor.

Craig puts his hands over his ears.

"Hard to predict our futures, isn't it Craig?" I say. "Some of us retire to places like the Bellemont—trade our desk chairs for wheelchairs."

"I hope I don't end up here," Craig says.

"Most of us don't," I say. "But we sure fear that we will."

"Here's a bed jacket you might want to wear," Bev says. She's a counselor and knows when to change a conversation. She holds up a rosy jacket, still on its hanger in its cleaner's bag. "Sometimes it feels good to get dressed up. Here's a book you might enjoy." She hands me *Colonel Pettigrew's Last Stand.* I am amused by the title, having had *my* last stand for a while. She and Craig take seats by the window-side of my bed. This is the first time I have spent time alone with the two of them.

I promise Craig that someday he and I will have a conversation about postmodernism, but now we converse about children, second marriages, weddings. Bev's story about her first wedding dress goes on for a while, as Southerners' stories often do, but all the while Craig is looking at her with total devotion. A surge of love for Bev overwhelms me. "I love you, Bev," I say, squeezing her hand. She kisses my cheek.

"I am Kiendra." A beautiful African woman is standing next to my bed. A hair-braid winds three times around the top of her head, held in place with a strip of Mali cloth. On her ring finger is an almond-size diamond. "I am you nurse. I check you in, now."

I look at the wall clock. Two a.m.

"Let me see you skin."

"My skin?"

"Yes. I need to look if you have sores."

"I don't."

"No, you don't," Kiendra says, after peering at my front side, back-side, and underside. "Now, I give you T.B. skin test."

She pricks my arm.

"Take these now. You meds."

"Isn't it a little late to take a Restoril?" I ask.

"Then don't take it," Kiendra says, and leaves.

"Please close the door," I yell. Too late.

A man's plaintive voice comes wailing down the corridor every thirty-seconds, "Help me . . . help me."

January 6

"Good morning, Laurel." A baritone voice. A smiling man with bright blue eyes stands at the foot of my bed. "I am Dr. Miller." He looks and sounds like Dr. Marcus Welby. A smiling blonde with purple eyeshadow stands next to him. She holds a clipboard. She looks like Joan Rivers. *Am I awake?*

It is 5:30 in the morning.

"I'm Kathy. *His* nurse." She beams with pride. *Is Dr. Miller her son, the doctor?* "You get both of us!"

"So, how are you feeling?" Dr. Miller asks.

"Tired," I say.

"Any pain?"

"Just some throbbing at my ankle."

"Dr. Girard did a lot on you," Dr. Miller says, looking at my chart. "Let's see . . . ninety–minutes—that's a long time—Hmm—excision of tibia, repair of torn tendon and stretched ligaments—Hmm—bruised nerves—cleaning up debris—Hmm . . . A lot."

"A lot," Kathy seconds.

"Skiing accident?" Dr. Miller asks.

"No," I say, surprised that I look like I might be a skier, albeit an injured one. "Nearly two years ago, an impatient traveler at O'Hare airport flung his suitcase off the rounder, hitting my ankle, and then, eighteen months ago, my ankle gave way on the Buckeye trail." *Poor Ernest felt so bad that he couldn't catch me before I fell.*

"You had physical therapy, though?" Dr. Miller notes.

"Yes, with my sports medicine doctor—but the physical therapy only made my instability, swelling, and pain worse. I got referred to Dr. Girard."

Dr. Girard's office was festooned with framed testimonials from the Blue Jackets hockey players and The Ohio State University's football players. I sat on a matted table, my shoes and socks off, when a small man with an enormous smile came bursting in with an entourage—interns? Residents? Definitely, a nurse in the pink scrubs.

"I'm Dr. Girard," he said in a French Canadian accent. "I've looked at your MRI and X-rays, Laurel. May I call you 'Laurel?' "

"Yes," I said. "And meet my husband, Ernest."

They shake hands the way men do, easily, sizing-up each other.

"You have three options, Laurel," Dr. Girard said, pointing to a wall-chart. "You can wear a brace the rest of your life and restrict your active life style. Or you can live in a wheelchair. Or you can get ankle surgery."

"How long is the recovery from surgery?" Ernest asked.

"It might take a year or eighteen months to fully recover," Dr. Girard said, exuding confidence.

I signed up for the surgery.

When the time approached, I reneged. I was too exhausted. "You're exhausted because of your ankle," Dr. Girard said. "Because you have a virus," my internist said. "Because you are going through a major life change—one that happens only once in a lifetime," my horoscope reader said, "and not one that everyone goes through." My subconscious said *Tsk-Tsk.* Whatever the reason, for a year I was chronically fatigued. Too tired for surgery. I began alternative therapies—homeopathic remedies and acupuncture. I thought I was healed.

"Look at the new X-ray, Laurel," Dr. Girard said, exuding bonhomie on my next visit, a year later. "Normally, I don't recommend surgery for anyone for anything, but I recommend it for you. The risks are few, the outcomes excellent. And, you are fortunate that you have not developed bone-spurs—yet."

"So, you've decided to get the surgery, after all," Dr. Girard's scheduler said, handing me a sheaf of papers to sign.

"Can I have the surgery in January?" I asked, preferring inactivity during the winter months. *A season for hibernation . . .*

"January 4th is open. Five weeks away."

"Okay."

"Did you know that Dr. Girard had the same surgery six weeks ago?" she said.

"What? No, I didn't."

"Tore his tendon skiing."

My anxiety rose. "Will he be able to operate on me?"

"He'll be fine. You'll be fine. It's made him more empathetic."

"Laurel?" The nurse Kathy's voice. "Are you with us?"

"Hmm. Oh, yes."

"You must hurt a lot," Kathy says, air-patting my wrapped-up ankle.

"Not really."

"I had the same surgery," Dr. Miller says, "so I know what you're going through. I'll order you stronger pain medicine."

I am thinking it is a good omen that both Drs. Miller and Girard have had *my* surgery.

"Please close the door," I say.

"I will. Go back to sleep, Hon," says Nurse Kathy. She and Dr. Miller leave to her hummings of Brahms's *Lullaby*.

"Help me . . . Help me" wails are deadened.

It is 6:00 a.m.

I have fallen back asleep.

"These you morning meds," Nurse Kiendra says, waking me and handing me a little plastic cup overflowing with pills. Normally, I only take three pills, all for my thyroid.

"What are all these?" I ask.

"They for you."

"What are they?"

"I will have to check. I take them away with me."

"Thank-you."

It is 6:30. I am asleep.

Knock-knock.

"Who's there?"

"I've brought your newspaper." An old man's voice. He comes into my room, uninvited, and drops the newspaper on my table.

At 6:50 Kiendra returns, waking me.

"These you morning meds," she says, handing me again the plastic cup overflowing with pills. "Doctor Miller's orders."

I recognize my thyroid pills, and I take those.

"Which is the antibiotic?" I ask.

Kiendra picks out a large yellow pill. She has magenta-colored nails.

"The pain pill?"

Kiendra picks out a blue one.

"I'll take those two," I say, as if I am ordering donuts. "But I don't want the others, whatever they are."

"Then don't take them."

"Time for your breakfast, Miz Laurel." A West-African woman's lilting voice. "I am Vena, your morning nurse's aide."

It is 7:30.

On my tray are orange juice, coffee, cow's milk, and some kind of hot oatmeal cereal that looks like throw-up.

"I can't eat this food," I say, gagging from its smell. Once when I stayed overnight at my Aunt Dorothy's she made me sit at the breakfast table until I had eaten my oatmeal. I sat there for hours, not eating. And then I threw up.

"Should I take the food away?" Vena asks.

"Yes, but please leave the coffee."

"Do you want to get dressed, now?"

"No."

"If you need me, push the call button," Vena says, taking out my tray and leaving my door open. I hear the cacophony of the prescription cart, food trays, the *Today Show,* staff shouting-out "Mornin" to one another, the "Help me… Help me" wails of the dementia resident, cries of despair, and a snorter-gagger-snot swallower in a wheelchair outside my open door. I push the call button.

"Did you need something?" A disembodied voice asks from the hallway. It is 8:00.

"Yes," I shout. "Please close my door."

"Hel-lo, Mis-sus Richerson." A Kentucky-accent. It is 8:40. I have had a little nap. A heavy-set woman in dark blue scrubs is beside my bed. She has such a pretty smile. "Gittin' some shut-eye?"

"Trying to."

"Ahm Effie Lou… Mayn't I call you 'Laurel'? "

I nod. She can call me "Beelzebub" for all I care.

"Ahm your occupational therapist. Are y'all ready to go to the Therapy Room?"

I nod. The sooner the therapy starts, the sooner I will be stronger, but, then again, I'm so tired.

"How's 'bout puttin' these on?" Effie Lou asks, taking a pair of gray jersey pants from my closet.

I shake my head. No pants are wide enough to go on over my foot-wrapping. "I'll just wear the pink fleece robe I bought especially for being in here. I bought it at CVS. It cost $10.00." *My tongue seems to be awake, even if my brain isn't.*

"Ahm glad there's a wheelchair here," she says. "We've plumb run out of 'em." Effie Lou lifts me into the wheelchair, which must have arrived during the night, adjusts the foot-thingamajigs. I am now a part of the clatter.

"Close my door, please, Effie Lou," I say.

Effie Lou pushes my chair toward the Therapy Room. At the nurses' station, two nurses are writing on residents' charts. The facility's records aren't computerized yet. A third nurse is on the phone, her back turned to the hallway. Getting out of his wheelchair is a handsome octogenarian. His alligator purse has fallen open on the floor. I can see his money. Three dollars. Next to his wheelchair is a little table set with playing cards, a newspaper, poker chips, and a child's wooden peg toy.

"Sit down, Trevor," Effie Lou orders. "Before you fall."

"Who is it?" Trevor asks. "I can't see you." His glasses are on the top of his head.

"It's me, Effie Lou. I have Laurel!"

"Hi, Trevor," I say. "I'm Laurel!"

Trevor sits back into his wheelchair and looks expectantly at me. "Can you help me find my room?" His voice is sweet.

"He cain't be in his room by hisself," Effie Lou whispers to me. To Trevor, she says, "It's not ready yet."

"Oh. It's not ready yet," Trevor repeats.

"Y'all have to wait here, Trevor," Effie Lou says. She picks up his purse and puts it on his lap.

"Okay. Thanks."

"Shouldn't he be strapped into his chair?" I ask Effie Lou

"Against the law to restrain them," Effie Lou says.

Trevor gets up again. Effie Lou shakes her head. He is not her responsibility. The nurses continue their recording and phone-calling. How demoralizing it must be for the nurses to work here where bureaucratic demands and terminal illnesses trump their original altruistic dreams and desires.

Effie Lou wheels me across an intersecting hallway, past the Bellemont's Administrative Offices to the Therapy Room. Several other patients are in the room. "Hi," I say, to nobody in particular. Twenty therapists work here, and that is why I chose this facility over a smaller, more intimate one slightly closer to home. I am privileged in having health insurance that gave me this choice. Here, I will have an hour or two of therapy six days a week. Occupational therapists will work on my torso and arms, and physical therapists on my hips and legs. Effie Lou hands me two two-pound weights and a Xerox copy of arm exercises—arms over head, side-lift arms, bicep curls, wrist twists. She sits down next to me on a roll about stool and watches me workout. I am very familiar with these exercises, having practiced them for years.

"Where are you from?" I ask Effie Lou, even though I am absolutely certain it is Kentucky.

"Johnson Holler—over yonder a patch," she answers. "Kin-tuc-ky!" We both laugh.

"My husban' sez he caint unnerstan' me," she continues hamming it up, accenting her accent.

"My husband's from southern Indiana," I say. "I can't always understand him either."

"How long you two bin married?" she asks.

"Thirty-two years," I say. "And you?"

"Two weeks. Wanna see the honeymoon pictures?"

"I do!" I say.

Effie Lou takes out her iPhone. Husband Tony is tall, dark, and handsome. They married at sunset on Miami Beach. He is wearing black pants and a collarless black shirt, and she is wearing a strapless white bridal gown. There are no witnesses. I tell her I am impressed. And I am. I am impressed with how this decade's "in" wedding ceremony is at sunset on a beach, the bride in white strapless, the groom in black, family and friends absent. The focus is on the bridal couple, the photo-ops for the memories, the "wedding" as "honeymoon." It never ceases to amaze me that doing what your peer-group does, no matter who they are or how young or old you are, does not feel imitative, common, or derivative, but special, unique, and even original, as you put your own spin—an A-line dress, lilacs, purple cummerbund—on the occasion. How empowered we feel when we successfully negotiate traditional acts (like getting married) in emergent cultural formats (the couple alone on the beach), tweaking them to please us (purple cummerbund), simultaneously *belonging* and *inventing*.

"Your first wedding?" I ask.

"Mine. Hiz second."

I think about my first wedding. Herb and I were both graduate students in Boulder, he in math and I in sociology. In the evening of my first day of graduate school, I heard a recording of a late Beethoven Quartet wafting down Haggerty Hall's corridor. I followed the music to Herb's office. Soon, we were surreptitiously sharing an apartment. The Dean of Women called me in. "You have a choice," she said. "Drop out of graduate school or get married. Your behavior has besmirched the reputations of all the Lady Buffs." Herb was not called in by the Dean of Men. He had not besmirched the men, the "Buffaloes." This was 1959. Herb was the only man I had dated who accepted my desire to have a career and children.

For our wedding, Herb bought a new gray suit, and I made a blue taffeta Audrey Hepburn-ish kind of dress. When stitching the final seam, I ran the sewing machine needle through the index finger of my left hand. I slipped my right hand under it to catch the blood, keep it off the dress, as if I were a bride-to-be in a Grimm's Fairy Tale. We were married in Chicago at the Edgewater Beach Hotel by a Jewish judge, honoring both my mother's Jewish background and my father's legal career. The judge concluded the ceremony by saying, "I condemn you to a happy life." There was a sit-down dinner reception for several hundred, mostly relatives, dreadful serenades by an accordion player, and dancing—the Jewish hora and Irish quadrilles. I got smashed on champagne. We stayed the night in the honeymoon suite. Late the next day, we packed our wedding gifts into our Morris Minor and drove to Chicago's south side to spend the night at my maid-of-honor's apartment before driving back to Colorado. During the night, the Morris Minor was broken into and our wedding presents were stolen.

For my second marriage—and last!—I had luscious burgundy-colored silk velvet made into a mandarin collared jacket and floor-length skirt. Under the jacket I wore a high-necked antique-white blouse. Ernest wore a dark blue suit and a designer tie. We had met ten years earlier in an encounter group at a Unitarian-Univeralist church retreat, the summer before my divorce. Ernest and I talked about the university, writing, and families. After his wife took off with another woman and he got divorced, he made a list of the women he wanted to date. There was only one name on it: Mine. Verta and Leila, friends of ours, gave us their house for the wedding and reception. Celeste, the facilitator of the encounter group and a recently ordained minister, married us. Roger, a friend and retired Lutheran minister, gave the blessing. Lots of friends came. My then twenty-year old son Ben talked physics to our friend, the logistics engineer. My sixteen year-old son Josh, recently sober, poured the champagne. Ernest's three daughters didn't come. My brother and brother-in-law didn't come. My sister came. Ernest's mother came and was scandalized by my red bridal dress. Ernest's Aunt Clona came. She gave us a paring knife and a butcher knife saying, "The knives you already have are too dull." This was 1981.

"I've been married twice," I say to Effie Lou. I don't say, *Second marriages are the triumph of hope over experience*, a Samuel Johnson aphorism I cross-stitched on linen. It hangs in our kitchen, near the round oak table.

"Hi, I'm Colleen." A strong-looking middle-aged woman joins us. She walks from side-to-side as if she has sea legs. "I'm your physical therapist," she says with a certitude that goes with her red hair.

"I'm ready," Effie Lou says, her accent diminished. She wheels me over to a pair of parallel bars, set at elbow height and puts a gait belt around my waist. Colleen instructs me to put weight on my "good leg," bend my "bad" leg back, and hold onto the parallel bars for balance. She holds the tail of the gait belt in one hand and my shoulder in the other. The wheelchair is in a locked position behind me. I can feel it with my calf, the way I was taught to feel for a chair when I was a teen in modeling-school and earning a little money as a department store model until my father nixed it saying it was a "seedy" occupation, controlled by mobsters. He nixed my dating a policeman, too, saying they were violent and corrupt.

"I can't put any weight on my left foot," I whine.

"I know. Don't worry," Colleen says. "I won't let that happen."

This parallel bar stuff is new to me, and I am fearful. I have no confidence in myself. What if I fall? What if I do put my bad foot down? Will I have to have the surgery again? I don't like putting my body at risk—I don't like not knowing how risky it is. It feels so risky. *Would I be yelled at if I did it wrong? Hurt myself?* I would feel so much more confident if I saw someone else doing this, first. I am a mimic. Always have been, always will be.

When I was perhaps three or four, my father would ask each guest to say something—anything. After they had all said whatever they wanted to say, I would go from guest to guest repeating back, word for word, intonation-by-intonation what each one had said. I don't know if I was showing off or if Father was showing me off, but I do know that I was being trained and rewarded for remembering and repeating verbatim what I heard. *Copy-Cat* was a compliment.

"Laurel, you are doing just fine," Colleen says. She sounds like a coach.

"Ready to play volleyball?" Effie Lou asks. She is standing at the far end of the parallel bars. She taps a yellow balloon toward me. Standing on my right foot, I release my right hand's hold on the parallel bar and spike that balloon. My killer-shot. One doesn't forget how to ride a bike, no matter how many years pass, nor have I forgotten how to play volleyball. I played on the intermural team at the University of Chicago, a school not known for its athletes. In my last volleyball game, the Woman's Army Corps' B-team (maybe F-team?) humiliated us. Me. Twenty-one to zero. Twice.

"Bring on the balloon!" I announce to Effie Lou. "I am an athlete!"

"Best balancer Ah've ever seen," says Effie Lou.

"And risk-averse," Colleen adds. "That's good. Now, let's have you do five-minutes on the NuStep—right foot only. Then, I'll wheel you on back."

Nearly fifty years ago, I had a Post-Doctoral Fellowship at Ohio State University's Inpatient Rehabilitation Center. My research question was "Who gets better?" What were then surprising statistical results, "getting better" was correlated with educational level, social-skills, post-rehab goals *and* how much the staff *liked* the patient. Liking, in turn, depended upon how societally valuable the staff perceived the patient to be and how compliant the patient was to the demands of therapy. Doing research in the rehab setting was difficult for me.

Patients assumed I was a "real" doctor and would ask me for medical advice or ask me to adjust a wheelchair lever or check a bandage. Sometimes, I found myself on the edge of practicing medicine without a license; always, I found myself not on the edge but smack in the middle of practicing emotional therapy—actively listening—before ethnographers admitted to doing such. Most of the inpatients were young men injured in car, diving, or other male, risky-behavior/work accidents. When I was asked to renew my post-doc the following year, I declined. I had one son, Ben, and was pregnant with another. I could not emotionally handle a career in medical sociology and motherhood.

Now, as I am wheeled away from my rehab Therapy Room, I take stock. Good that I am educated, have social-skills, and post-rehab goals. Better to work hard, do as I'm told, and to stay risk-averse. Best to have the staff like me.

"Keep up the good work," Colleen says.

"Hi, Trevor," I say. "It's me, Laurel."

"Can you show me the way out?" he asks.

"You have to wait here," I say.

He looks agitated.

It is 10:15. The nurses are doing paperwork.

Colleen wheels me into my room, and teaches me how to pivot and transfer from the wheelchair to my bed. My first little bit of independence. "See you about the same time tomorrow," she says, side-stepping out the door.

The nurses' aide Vena comes in and puts several pillows under my left foot and re-attaches my DonJon IceMan. She hums *Amazing Grace* as she leaves.

Snort. Grunt. Spit. The choking woman in the wheelchair is parked at my door.

"Vena, close the door, please," I say.

Too late.

"Hi, can I come in?" A buxom forty-ish woman in a wheelchair is at my door, now. She's wearing a loose fitting T-shirt, no bra and black shorts.

"Sure," I say, glad that the snorter has wheeled away.

"I'm Renee. I'm your across the hall neighbor. Room 113. " Her hair is dark, long, and wavy. Her eyes are hazel, her skin clear. She looks like Jane Russell.

She gives a deep chortle and wheels close to my bed. Her right leg has been amputated above the knee, the left leg below. The right one dangles over her seat. Both stumps are bare.

"I'm Laurel."

"Your name is on your door."

"So much for privacy rights, huh?"

Renee chortles again and gives me an appraising look. "You're the one with those dogs, aren't you?" she asks. She seems to be waving her legs, thumping them up and down, adjusting her catheter. She extends her neck and retracts it.

"Yes. Bashi and Lily. Papillons. We gave them their forever homes."

"Do you think they could visit me?" Renee asks in a husky voice.

"They'd love it," I say. "They're learning to be therapy dogs."

Renee asks why I am here and I tell her about my ankle surgery—which seems so trivial when I look at her. She tells me she has been in the Bellemont for three months, having been sent here from Eastward Orthopedic Clinic in Pittsburgh because they couldn't do anything more for her, and having been sent there by Jefferson Hospital in Youngstown because they couldn't do anything for her at all. She had been in Jefferson for a heart stent. The cardiologist decided to go in through her groin.

"He hit my stomach aorta and all the 'crap' went down to my legs," she tells me.

"Oh, Renee."

"My daughter had to decide right then whether to let me die or get my legs amputated. She's twenty-two. What does she know?" Renee takes a handkerchief from her shorts' waistband, wipes her eyes.

"I am so sorry," I say. I don't know what else to say.

"See you later," Renee says, wheeling herself out. She pulls her head down until her shoulders rise above her ears. Her wheelchair is her carapace.

I don't shout at her to close the door.

It is 11:00.

"Yes, you can pet them." Ernest's voice down the hallway.

Jingle-jangle.

"Going to see Laurel." Ernest's voice closer to my room.

"Yap."

"Yap."

"Oh! Dogs!" I hear Trevor's voice.

"You can pet them." Ernest's voice. "Bashi and Lily."

"Thank you." A smoker's voice.

Jingle-jangle.

"They're friendly." Ernest's voice even closer.

"Pretty puppies!" A child's voice.

"Yap."

"Yap."

"They're Papillons. You can pet them . . . You can touch their ears."

Grunt . . . snort. That woman parked outside my door again.

"Bring them over later, huh? Room 113." Renee's seductive voice.

Then the pups dance into my room, up on their hind legs, going around in circles, nipping each other's cheeks, yapping their little yaps. "Oh hurrah!" they seem to be saying, "Laurel's here! We found her!!" Ernest puts them on my bed. Bashi stretches out on my chest, like a little heating pad. Lily guards my foot. I tell Ernest about my eventful morning, and then the dogs and I take a dog-nap.

"Your lunch, Miz Laurel," the West African aide, Vena, says, putting a tray on my little-swing-away-table. It is noon. "Those your dogs?" Vena backs away.

"They're nice dogs," I say.

"I don't like dogs much," she says, backing away farther.

I read a lot about dogs before we got Bashi and Lily. I know that dogs in Africa are often feral and rabid, and when traveling in packs they are formidable. If a dog lives in a village, you own it by letting it sleep in your yard. Never inside. Dogs are not pets. They have no names. I watched a video clip of an American teacher bringing her pet bulldog mix into a classroom in Ghana. The children screamed in fright, ran for cover. They cannot believe that the teacher is putting a treat into a dog's mouth and that the dog has not bitten her hand off.

"My dogs don't bite," I say to Vena. "They aren't like African dogs." But, then, I think, it is probably not only African dogs that might scare Vena, but American dogs, too. She might very well live in a neighborhood populated with guard dogs—Pit bulls, Dobermans, German Shepherd mixes. Those dogs scare me, too. *My privileged life is showing.*

"You can pet these dogs," I say.

"Leave it be," Ernest says, giving me a warning look that I ignore. I think my dogs have the ability—charms and looks—to ease people's fears, bring comfort, to make friends. Am I being arrogant? Am I putting my own desires above the fears of my West African nurses' aide?

I find a way to compromise.

"You don't have to pet them," I say. "But they would like it."

Vena comes closer and tentatively touches Lily's head. Lily doesn't bat an eyelash. Vena seems proud of herself. She is standing taller. It is probably the first time in her life that she has touched a dog.

"She's soft," Vena says.

"Her name is Lily," I say.

"Bye, Lily," Vena says as she leaves. "Call if you need something, Miz Laurel."

"Let's see what you have for lunch." Ernest takes the green plastic cover off the plate. "Looks like mystery meat—and beans—and noodles."

"Do you want it?" I ask. The smell gags me.

"Maybe the dogs will like it," Ernest suggests after a tasting of his own. He turns the green cover into a water-bowl, and sets the plate down next to it. The dogs turn their noses up at the food but lap away at the water.

I eat the gluten-free crackers and applesauce I had brought from home.

"I bet the dogs would like going to the ersatz dog park," I say, pointing out my window to the enclosed courtyard.

"Outside?" Ernest says to the dogs—their cue word to get ready to "get busy."

From my bed, I can see them running around, romping in the snow, chasing each other's tails, digging away. Lily has unearthed a bone. It looks like a femur. Ernest takes it away. A gray-haired woman wrapped in a blanket sits in her wheelchair in the covered patio. A nurses' aide is beside her. Both are smoking.

A nurse comes in to dispense my mid-day meds, Vena takes away my lunch tray and asks after Lily, and a perky activities manager Penny invites me to the bingo game. I fall asleep.

"I brought the dogs to see your neighbor Renee in 113," Ernest says.

"Hmm?" I say.

"I'm sorry. Did I wake you?"

"That's okay, Ernest," I mumble. "I'm glad you're here."

"Lily sat on Renee's lap for twenty minutes. Renee didn't want to put her down."

"And Bashi?"

"He curled up beside her wheelchair."

"Hmmm."

"Renee has quite a story," Ernest says. "Double-amputee. I feel terrible for her."

"Me, too…hmmmm."

"I'll take the dogs home now and come back this evening."

"Bring back rice milk and Rice-Chex, please."

"Sure."

"Hmm. Please close my door."

CHECK HALL 100 EXIT CHECK HALL 100 EXIT CHECK HALL 100 EXIT RRRRRRRRIIIIINNNNNGGGGGG RRRRRRRRIIIIINNNNNGGGGGG

"Hello. Laurel?" It is 1:30. A strawberry-blonde woman in a red dress has awoken me. "I'm Mira—I have to ask you some admissions questions."

"I want to sleep," I say.

"I'll come back later, then. What say in twenty-minutes?"

Ring-ring-ring.

"Hello."

"Hi, Laurel. How are you feeling?"

"Okay."

"Oh, did I wake you? I'll call back later."

Who was that masked caller?

Knock-knock.

"Who's there?" I ask.

"Respiratory therapy."

"I don't have that."

"Sorry."

Knock-knock.

"Come in."

"Mail. Oh, no. Wrong room."

"Okay."

"Wait. These flowers are for you."

"Hi again, Laurel. It's Mira from admissions."

It is 1:50.

"It won't take long," she says. "Do you want to sit at the table?"

I want to say, *Are you crazy or just not observant or have you not read your own admissions work?* But I just shake my head and point to my wrapped foot.

Mira pulls a chair up to my bedside and takes a several inch-thick stack of papers from her briefcase. I listen, sort of, and sign away my life savings. Maybe. Probably not. Probably Medicare covers it all. She puts a purple folder on my table with my copies, thanks me and leaves. It is 2:10. I push my call button.

Vena comes in at 2:40. She helps me to the bedside commode. She asks after Lily.

"Hello, Laurel." A young man's voice. It is 3:00. "I am Brandon."

I appraise the tall, dark, nervous-looking stranger at my door. He is twentyish, tall, well-scrubbed and dapperly dressed in a dark blue suit that looks new, a light blue shirt and blue-striped tie. Not exactly a romance-novel hero.

"Your tie and shirt look very good together, Brandon," I say. I enjoy complimenting men on their sartorial choices. When I do so, their chests expand, they cock their heads, and look pleased. As commenting on any student's clothing when I was a professor could be interpreted as "sexual harassment" because of the power-differential, I never complimented my students on their clothing choices. But here in the Bellemont, because I am "disempowered," I am "empowered" to take notice, comment and make a guy feel good about himself.

"Thanks," Brandon says, broadening his chest. "They came together. As a set." He stands near the door, lifting his feet up and down like a colt. "I'm from the business office," he continues. "How is everything? Can I do anything for you?"

"Ask me tomorrow, but not today," I say.

I fall back asleep.

At 4:00, the nurses' aide Jamal comes in and awakens me. He looks at my wall clock, adjusts his wrist-watch. He looks jittery.

"I have to weigh you," he says. "You have to be weighed before you're here twenty-four hours. I'm a little late, but..."

"I can't stand up," I say.

"I was supposed to do it yesterday, but . . ."

"I can't stand up," I repeat.

"I know," Jamal is pacing the room, fiddling with his glasses. "I have to take you in the wheelchair to the weighing station. Weigh you in the wheelchair and then . . ." Jamal stops talking as he helps me pivot from the bed to the chair. He pushes me down the hallway and onto a ramp with a scale. I feel as if I am a chunk of meat in a basket, and I am afraid that my left foot will bang into the scale-pole.

"Have you weighed people before?" I ask.

"First time," he says. He flashes a grin. "Does 212 pounds sound right?"

"Try 165."

"Okay," he says. "I'd guesstimate the chair weighs forty-seven pounds, then."

"You're good at math," I comment, as Jamal wheels me back to my room. "And I think you know French, too."

"Yes. I've had three years of pre-med. School work is easy but I have a character flaw—I procrastinate." Jamal smiles, then laughs and guffaws. I laugh, too. His jitteriness is gone.

"My granddaughter procrastinates some, too," I say. "Less now, that she has found work she wants to do."

"I get that," Jamal says. "I realized I didn't want to be a doctor. My parents wanted it."

"But you still want to be in the medical field?" I ask.

"Maybe . . . I don't know . . . This job was available . . . I could live at home."

"How old are you?"

"I just turned twenty-one."

"Lots of living ahead of you, Jamal."

Ring ring ring.

"Hello."

"Ernest called and told us you are doing fine." My older brother Barrie's voice. He lives in Shreveport, Louisiana. As a little boy, he was shy and introverted. To build his confidence, and "bring him out,"

Father introduced him to doing magic tricks. Barrie took to it and was on the *Kukla, Fran, and Ollie Show* when he was a pre-teen. He sawed me in half. White rabbits and gray doves lived peacefully together on our back porch. Now, he's a retired professor of economics and a member of the exclusive Magic Circle in London. He travels the world teaching elite magicians his tricks.

"Are you in pain?" he asks.

"No."

"That's good. You sound tired."

"I am."

"Keep getting well. I'll call tomorrow, Honey."

Ring ring ring.

"Hi, Ho-nee."

"Hi, Ellyn!"

Ring ring ring.

"Hello."

"Hi, Laurie." My college roommate's alto voice.

"Nora, hi."

Ring ring ring.

"Hi Mom."

"Hi Josh."

Ring ring ring . . .

Ring ring ring . . .

My older son Ben and his wife Tami come into my room, bearing gifts: Fresh flowers in a blue curvy vase, and dinner, Japanese noodles from Noodles. They settle in the window-side chairs. It is 5:30. Both of them are blond, blue-eyed, and trim. He is nearly a foot taller than she. If I hadn't seen Ben being born, I would have doubted he was mine. No brown eyes or a lick of brown hair. Ben's coloring favors his father, Herb, but his athletic build, strength, and stamina favor my father.

Tami is a radiographer at the Veteran's Administration, the only medical person in our family. She loves her work. Ben is an electronic engineer/software developer, the only person at his job who knows the old system, the new system, and the in-between systems. He has an office with a window near the "help-desks," as those helpers often need his help. When they are not at work, Ben and Tami are riding their bikes, fixing up their house, or planning additions to it. They live a mile south of me. They've have been married twenty-two years, and they still act like newlyweds. I am surprised that Tami isn't sitting on Ben's lap right now.

"How are you feeling, Laurel?" Tami asks.

"So, what have you been doing?" Ben asks. This is his stock question.

"Shana sends her love," Tami says. Shana is their daughter. She has a job she loves—exhibit developer at the Minnesota Science Museum. Two years ago, I took Shana to France. We liked Paris, but fell in love with the village of Roussillon in Provence. The village is settled beside ochre cliffs, and its houses mirror the extraordinary range of colors in those cliffs. It reminded me of Sedona. I bought natural pigments there for Ernest. He is a prolific painter. Shana and I spent hours in a little craft store, until Shana decided on a pattern for an 18th century Provencal dress. Someday, she may make it. If Ernest and I had had a child, she would be Shana's age.

Jingle-jangle.

Ernest comes in with the dogs who give dog-kisses to Tami and Ben, before settling on my bed.

"You can sit here, Ernest," Tami says. She gives up her chair to sit on Ben's lap.

We have our normal conversation—about Ben's work, Tami's work, their house, Tami's sisters, Shana. I feel grateful that I have this good relationship with them, that there is no "elephant" in the room. I am grateful that my son Ben has this good life. That these two found each other.

"OMG, it's 8:00!" Tami says. "We didn't mean to tire you out."

"Anything we can get you?" Ben asks.

"I've got it pretty well covered," Ernest answers, pointing to the Rice Chex.

"The rice milk can go in the nurses' refrigerator," I say.

"Are you sure?"

"Yes. I asked."

CHECK HALL 100 EXIT CHECK HALL 100 EXIT CHECK HALL 100 EXIT RRRRRRRIIIIINNNNNGGGGGG RRRRRRRIIIIINNNNNNGGGGGG

"Ben and Tami didn't know about the code," Ernest says.

"Ben will have fun talking about the robot-voice," I say. "He'll probably have an Einsteinium level explanation of how it works. Or a way to improve upon it." I find myself thinking about Ben as a toddler. His favorite toy was a wind-up phonograph. He'd put different objects on the turn table, spin it at different speeds, and speculate, I thought, about centrifugal force. He would be entertained on long car trips with his car-book, *The Way things Work*. He spent hours studying the diagrams.

"I'm feeling a little melancholic," I say to Ernest.

"It's probably the meds," he says.

"Hello, Laurel." Nurse Kiendra is at the door.

"Here are you nighttime meds," she says.

She hands me a little plastic cup with only three pills.

"I'll take the sleeping pill a little later," I say.

"Do as you wish but promise not you sell it."

"Will you put my rice-milk in the refrigerator, please?"

Kiendra takes out a wide Sharpie and writes "Laurel #112" on the carton. She takes it, smiles at Ernest, and leaves.

"Time for us to leave, too," Ernest says, gathering up Lily and Bashi.

Jingle-jangle.

It is 9 p.m. I find "Project Runway" on the TV. At 10:00, I take my sleeping pill and then release my silver Tibetan healing balls from their black velvet bag, a gift twenty-years ago from my far-away friend, Susan. Their sound is soothing.

January 7

There will be a rhythm to my mornings, of this I am already certain. The newspaper delivery at too early an hour, the nurse bringing me more medicines than I want, the inedible breakfast tray, the rancid smell of steamed food and the clinical smell of Clorox, the nurse's aide helping me with my morning toilette, the cacophony of the metal-against-metal of the serving cart, the shout-outs of staff to each other, the moans, snorts and the "help me . . . help me" of residents, my shouting, "Close the door, please!" Occupational and physical therapy. Sweet anticipation of Ernest, Lily and Bashi, the loveliness of flowers in my room, and out my window witnessing the sky kiss the earth.

"Ready for physical therapy?" Colleen asks. Her side-to-side listing is more severe today. "How do you feel?" She helps me pivot out of bed into my wheelchair and puts a gait-belt around my waist.

"I thought gait belts weren't allowed?" I say, and immediately feel sorry that my question implicitly criticizes Colleen.

"P.t.s can restrain residents," she says. "So they'll be safe when we work them. Nurses aren't allowed to, though."

"So lots of restraints on the nurses, huh?" I say.

"Let's go," Colleen says.

I feel as if I have inadvertently gotten on the wrong side of Colleen today.

She wheels me down the hall.

"Hi, Trevor," I say. He's in his wheelchair by the nurses' station. He's wearing blue pin-striped pajamas and is "reading" the *Dispatch*.

"Who is it?" he says. "I don't have my glasses."

"It's me, Laurel. Looks like they found your room."

"Where's my room?" Trevor gets up.

"You have to wait, Trevor," Colleen says. "Sit down."

"Bye, Trevor," I say.

Colleen shakes her head.

"Is he always out in the hall?" I ask.

"He can't be left alone," Colleen says. "He gets up and could fall. He needs a private nurse." *I wonder what a private nurse costs?*

"Elaine?" I see my dear friend coming towards me. She's a nurse. Retired.

She air-hugs me and her deep blue eyes scan me. "I can't actually hug you," Elaine says "because I think I might be coming down with something." She gave me eye drops once. She scrubbed her hands, scrubbed my cheek, gently tipped my head back, lowered my eyelids, dripped the drops into my eyes, told me to close them and hold that position for thirty-seconds. I never had such care taken of my eyes before or since. Elaine is careful. Hmm. Full of Care. "But I wanted to *see* your facility and *see* you."

"Thanks." I air-hug her back.

"Looks good," she says. "Keep getting well."

Colleen and I arrive at the Therapy Room where Colleen supervises my leg and foot exercises. A nurse's aide wheels Trevor into the Therapy Room. "Can you watch him?" she asks.

Colleen mutters something like, *I've got my own work to do*, but hands him a wooden peg set. Trevor looks around at the Therapy Room equipment—parallel bars, raised mats, NuStep bikes. I wonder if he is remembering a time when he worked-out or ran long distances, and got massaged. He starts to get up. Colleen puts a gait belt around him. He looks so wistful. I just want to get up—which I can't do either—and give him a hug. I wonder if he ever gets touched.

"Laurel, you really look good." Suzanne is here! She reaches down and hugs me, and gives me a kiss on my cheek. She is wearing killer boots and a faux-mink jacket. She is letting her hair turn gray.

"Oh, Suzanne! So do you!!"

"Colleen," I say, "meet Suzanne…the mother of my grandson…hmm…my ex-daughter-in-law." Suzanne and my son Josh have been divorced for thirteen years.

"*Friend*," Suzanne says, a little embarrassed, I think.

"Special friend," I say. "Healer." Suzanne and I are friends. I love her. I am eternally grateful to her, not only for my grandson, but for introducing me to the world of alternative medicine. She helped me before my surgery by suggesting what homeopathic remedies I should use, foods to eat, exercises to avoid, and by sharing her own recovery story from shredded leg muscles, including her months in a wheelchair and on crutches.

"Pretty ring, Suzanne," I say,

"It was my grandmother's pearl and Glenn designed the setting," she says. Glenn is her fiancé. They were sweethearts in college. She had written him a letter wanting to "talk"; he thought she wanted to break up. He kept that letter for the next thirty-eight years.

"Have you set your wedding date?" I ask.

"We haven't sold our houses yet, and we want all the kids…"

"Laurel?" A muscle-bound woman with short-blond hair is calling my name. "I'm Rhonda, your occupational therapist today."

"Where's Effie Lou?" I ask.

"She had some trouble at home. So, Laurel, get up!"

'What? I'm not allowed to put any weight on my foot."

"I'll just help you get up."

"Did you read my chart?"

"No, I haven't had time. I just got here."

I stare at her.

"Don't look at me with those squirrely eyes," Rhonda says.

"Laurel might lack some confidence if you aren't familiar with her chart," Suzanne says in a most conciliatory and conflict-stopping manner. *I am so glad she is here.*

"Okay," Rhonda says. "Then you need to learn how to use your wheelchair by yourself."

She instructs me to push on the rubber wheel.

"I found it easier," Suzanne intervenes, "when I put my hands way back on the metal wheels, and pushed those."

"Whatever..." Rhonda says, rolling her eyes and her shoulders. "Okay, Laurel, transfer from the wheel chair to the NuStep."

I wheel away following Suzanne's instructions but I can't stop. The wheelchair continues to roll. Rhonda ignores Suzanne's warnings about how the situation is unsafe and extremely dangerous.

"The brakes aren't working," Suzanne says, pulling back on the wheelchair's arms.

"They're fine," Rhonda says, dismissively. "Laurel's just not doing it right."

"Let's go," Suzanne says wheeling me out of the Therapy Room to the nurse's station. She asks for a maintenance man and wheels me back to my room.

"Sorry, I have to leave," Suzanne says, giving me another hug and cheek-kiss. "I have to catch a flight to California."

In my room, there is a pretty young woman with soft wavy hair. Her light blue scrubs mean that she is a nurses' aide. I think she must be a Pisces, because she moves smoothly as if she is swimming under water. Maybe her eyes are on the side of her head, like a cuttlefish, because she seems to have taken in all corners of my room. The flowers have been deadheaded, my bedclothes changed, the bed table cleared of its detritus, my water pitcher refreshed. The long tails of her tunic move like fins. She shimmers.

"I'm Brooke," she says in a breathy voice, as if she misses being in the ocean. "Let me help you into bed, and set up your IceMan. Man, it's cool!"

I laugh at her little joke. I like her. "Do you like your work?" I ask.

"Actually, I do. I think of myself as being in customer relations." She notices the books on my table. "I like to read," she says. "Right now, I'm reading Margaret Atwood's *Surfacing.*"

"I met Atwood once," I say. I decide not to tell her the embarrassing story about Atwood and me at the Kentucky Women's Writing Conference. I had submitted my poem about lotioning my mother's legs the night before she died of cancer. Atwood chose it to Xerox and distribute to the several hundred workshop attendees. I was beside myself with pride until Atwood publicly picked the poem apart declaring it "not universal." "Atwood's a Queen Bee," a workshop attendee whispered in my ear. In the Seventies, believing rewards for women were severely rationed, queen bees buzzed about in women's spaces, stinging any potential competition. I still vacillate between anger and embarrassment when I think about Atwood, and I wish I were not thinking about her now. My mind seems to be wandering.

"My mind seems to be wandering," I say to Brooke.

"Probably the meds," she says.

"You have a wheelchair problem?" A Scandinavian-looking man is at the door. "I'm Gunther from maintenance."

I signal him to come in and to check out the chair.

"These brakes are completely shot," he says. "Nobody should be using this chair. I'll come back and fix them." I wonder why *this* wheelchair came to be in my room. I put a brake on my burbling paranoia.

"Here's a little pot of crocuses for you." My memoir-writing friend Linda R. has come into my room. She is scheduled for knee replacement surgery, and here she has hobbled down this long corridor to bring me a harbinger of spring. "I can't stay," she says. "But I wanted to give you a hug."

"Me, too!" Little Linda T., another memoirist, comes. "I brought you apples. You know, keep the doctor away."

"I'm just here for a few minutes," Cheryl says, coming into my room as my memoir-writing friends leave. "I've brought you your Christmas present!" Cheryl is a dear friend, a psychiatric nurse. Maybe I need her. I'm feeling odd. She's bundled up in her signature purple jacket, gloves, and Icelandic hat.

"Last year's or next year's?" I ask. Then I realize that Christmas was only a couple of weeks ago. It is early in January. *My grip on the calendar seems to be loosening.*

The gift is wrapped in purple-glittery paper with a little silver ornament upon which Cheryl has penned my name. "When I saw it, I knew it was for you." Cheryl beams. Inside the wrapping is a fleece blanket with Navajo patterns in Sedona colors.

"Perfect," I say.

"Everything's right where it's supposed to be," Cheryl says. This is her signature attitude towards life.

"Can I put it on the bed for you?" Brooke asks. Without waiting for an answer, she tidies me under the blanket.

"I've got the new brakes," Gunther is at the door. "All right if I fix the chair, now?"

I nod my assent.

"You're looking really good, Laurel," Cheryl says. It means a lot to me to hear her say that—I know that sounds trite, but it does mean a lot because she is a psychiatric nurse. She knows how good-healing-persons look, act, and sound.

"Am I?"

"All fixed," Gunther says. "Shouldn't give you any more trouble."

"I'll adjust the blind," Brooke says. "Get the sun out of your eyes."

"Call if you need anything," Cheryl says, leaving.

"Call if you need anything," Brooke says, leaving.

"Yap. Yap."

"Woof. Woof."

"Yap. Yap."

"He wants to be friends," I hear Ernest's voice over Bashi's yapping and some big dog's woofing.

"Bring Lily in here," Renee's voice, simultaneously sultry and imperious.

I fall into a sweet reverie, an inside quietness.

"Weren't you sitting at the table?" I ask Ernest. "When did you move to the window?"

"I've always been at the window," he says. "You were sleeping when I came in. You must have been dreaming."

I feel the warmth of Lily and Bashi along my legs, and I reach down to pet them. *Jingle-jangle.* Lily looks so compassionate with her brindle colored ears, tiny head, and kind eyes. Bashi looks regal, elegant in his black and white fur, ready for a formal bash. They cuddle into the fleece blanket, their fur coat colors blending right in.

Ernest tells me about his conversation with Renee. She works with a local contractor for the Federal Energy Department—or did, until they forced her to take retirement after her amputations. She has top security clearance and she's still waiting to be debriefed.

"Energy Department?" I am thinking of coal, gas, wind, and sun. "Why do they need top security?"

"They're in charge of our nuclear arsenal, Darlin'." Ernest shakes his head. "You know, hydrogen bombs, nuclear subs...plutonium enrichment...and who knows what else, now..."

I squirm and change the subject. "Did she hold Lily again?"

"She wanted to know how much she cost."

"You didn't tell her, did you?"

"No, I told her what we tell everyone, that they are rescued dogs."

They are rescued dogs in a way. We saved Bashi and Lily from lives as show-dog breeders. Lily had three different owners and three different names. Much of her life she spent in a kennel in a van being driven to dog shows in which she couldn't compete because she hadn't thrived enough to meet conformation standards. She weighed less than four pounds when we got her. Her littermate, Bashi, had been a novice champion in Canada, but because his left front foot turned out slightly, he would never be a champion in America and wasn't "finished." Both of our Paps were washed up, retired from the breeding pool, at fifteen months. We gave them their *forever homes.*

"What did Renee say?" I ask.

"Never seen a dog like Lily at the pound. And then she thumped her thighs with her thumbs."

"What adorable dogs!" Brooke has glided in with my lunch. "I can get another tray for them, if you want."

"They can have this one," I say.

"I can't eat the food here, either," she says, setting the plate on the floor. This time the Paps lap at the gravy-covered meat loaf and mashed potatoes.

"Do you want a tray?" Brooke asks Ernest.

"Hmm . . . no."

Brooke leaves, Paps nap, Ernest reads Faulkner on his Kindle and I— I— I?

"Here's your dinner, Laurel." Jamal has brought in my tray. He looks bigger and darker than I remember him. He smells musky.

"I don't know where the day went," I say.

"You've been sleeping." His voice sounds deeper than I remember it. He takes the cover off the plate.

"Yuck. It smells like rotten eggs."

Jamal chuckles—a loud chuckle—and covers the hot food back up. "Maybe you'd like to eat the cold fruit salad?"

I stab a fork in a piece of canned peach, and leave it there.

Now, it is 8:15 at night. I have pushed my call button. I am waiting. Waiting. Waiting.

I need the nurses' aide so I can use the bedside commode. I can feel Bashi against my right arm, under the blanket, and I can feel Lily under the blanket, curled up on my left leg. I can smell their doggy smell, like overripe cantaloupes—and musty, like Bluebird Cottage at Lake Bluestone. I reach down to pet Bashi, but he is not there. I push my call button again.

PUSH!

PUSH!

It is 8:30.

PUSH!

I feel Lily licking my leg. "Good little dog," I say and call her. But she doesn't come. She isn't there.

PUSH!

Bashi feels so warm and furry lodged under my armpit, and down my side. "I don't want to roll over on you, Bashi," I say. But he doesn't "yap" back; he doesn't utter a sound. I can't see him. He's not there.

PUSH!!!

It is 8:45.
I am very scared.
"Good dogs."

PUSH!!!!

It is 9:00. I am trapped in bed. *Can I figure out what to do?* Yes! I will phone Ernest.

"Hello, Darlin'," Ernest' s voice. "What's up?"

"I'm so scared."

"Why?"

"I am having phantom senses—tactile feelings. And phantom smells. I can feel and smell the dogs, but they aren't here. Are they?"

"They're here. In their kennels. Have you called your nurse's aide?"

"Forty-five minutes ago. She doesn't come."

"Try the front desk."

"There is no one there after 6:00."

"I'm driving over right now," Ernest says.

"Maybe I should call 911? I have to pee, too."

"I'll be right there sooner than the squad. You'll be okay. It's the Vicodin. It's giving you hallucinations."

"That's right. That's the word—ha-lu-ci-na-tions. "

"Did you want something, Miz Laurel?" Vena's West African lilting voice. "Ernest, Vena is here now."

"Are you sure she is *really* there?"

"Yes. She smells like pizza."

"I was having supper," Vena says. "For a half-hour."

"My call light was on for forty-five minutes!" I am in a rage. I want to punch her. "Why didn't you have someone sub for you?" *Malingerer!*

Vena looks down, starts to speak and doesn't.

"Help me to the commode," I order.

"Time for you meds," Nurse Kiendra says. I didn't see her come in. I think she is really here.

"Why didn't *you* answer my call light? *Malingerer!*"

"Not my job . . . I was busy."

"I'm not taking the Vicodin," I say, belligerently. I want to pull that blood-diamond right off her ring finger.

"You need for pain."

"No. I don't."

In the wee hours of the morning, I awaken, still pain-free. I know I am in bed in Room 112 in the Bellemont. I know there are no dogs in bed with me. The peat moss surrounding the crocuses is the room's only scent, Cheryl's fleece blanket the only warm thing touching me. I breathe deeply, breaths of relief. Gratitude overwhelms me. I am "me" again. How horrid it is to not know what is real and what is hallucination. How absolutely ghastly it would be to have apparitions, phantom touches, and smells enter your world willy-nilly. Day after day, year after year, decade after decade. To come and go as they wish. Some of them warning you of dangers, others preparing you to defend yourself. Not being able to trust your senses or your feelings. Living in anger or fear or anxiety or preparedness for whatever. Oh God! I had a single day of that—off and on—and less than an hour of severe hallucinatory experience. I cannot imagine what it would be like to live my whole life in that state of uncertainty, fear, and wrath. My empathy for people with schizophrenia is no longer just mental and moral; it has settled into my Being. I get why some choose suicide. I think I would.

Two of my friends' schizophrenic brothers have committed suicide this year. These friends, having lived through chaotic childhoods, fear for their children's sanity, their family's welfare. They question whether their children's behavior is normal for teenagers or harbingers of severe mental illness. They know there is no quick cure and that once their children turn eighteen they have no legal options. Every time a story hits the news about a homicidal rampage, they are anguished if they learn the perpetrator was an off-meds schizophrenic. One friend, whose son is living on the streets, says her "heart stops" until she reads the killer's name: not her son. When he was thirteen, my own son, Ben, told me he was "hearing a voice" telling him what to do. For that brief period, I struggled with what his life might be like and what my life would be like, if that were true. I still shudder remembering my angst, fear. I sought counseling for him. The voice, as it turned out, was his own voice, his conscience. He was talking to himself. How normal. How relieving.

&

CHAPTER 2

"We Don't Know Why, Yet"

January 8

"Sunday breakfast is always a little better," Brooke says in her breathy voice. Her wavy hair is escaping its net. She takes the cover off my breakfast tray with a flourish. "Voila! Bob Evans sausages… French toast… orange juice." Brooke glides to the window and raises the blind. "There. A nice sunny day for you!" She stands akimbo at the foot of my bed like a starfish, and asks, "How are you today, Laurel?"

"Much better," I say. "I've stopped taking the Vicodin. No more pain pills for me." I take a teensy bite of sausage. "Sausage is good," I say. I pour some maple syrup on the French toast and cut off a bite. "This is good, too. I am famished." I gobble all my food

"Don't you like orange juice?" Brooke asks, noting I haven't touched it.

"It is too acidic."

"What kind of juice do you like?"

"Cranberry."

"So does your neighbor, Renee."

"Are you usually here on Sunday mornings," I ask.

"I'm making up some lost time."

"You do a great job. Thanks."

"You're welcome." Brooke hesitates a moment, then says. "My mom called today and told me how proud she was of me."

"How are you doing, Laurel." Colleen, my p.t. is at my door. She is bouncing from foot-to-foot, trying to take the pressure off her back. "Ready?"

"I don't ever want to work with that horrid Rhonda again. She could have really messed—"

"There are personality differences. We try to make sure—"

"—me up bad. She hadn't—"

"—that therapists and clients are—"

"—even looked at my chart—"

"—compatible."

"—not to mention—"

"Not to worry. Effie Lou's back."

"And my wheelchair's brakes are fixed."

"Then we'll practice you doing the driving."

Colleen pivots me into the chair and pushes me into the hallway. Renee is in her wheelchair outside her door. Her amputation scars are red. She's crying.

"Hi, Renee," I say. "This is my first time to drive my chair."

"I can help you with that," she sniffs. "I've had lots of practice."

"See you later."

Colleen steers me toward the left side of the corridor. The snorting, gagging, snot-swallowing woman is parked on the right side, near my door. Why does she hang out by my door? Does she have lung problems and dementia?

I decide to give the Corridor Woman the story my Aunt Paulie, told me over and over about herself when she was 87, a nursing home resident with COPD and dementia:

> "Aren't I pretty? See my blue party dress." She thinks she's eight years old going to her friend Rosemary's birthday party. "I'll have cake. Ice Cream. I'll win Pin-the Tail-on-the-Donkey." She fiddles with her hospital smock. "I am waiting for Uncle Leif to drive me. Are you coming to the party, too?"

My brother-in-law Paul insisted on correcting Aunt Paulie, persistently telling her that she was an elderly woman in a nursing home. Somehow, he thought that shaking a reality stick at her would cure her dementia, or at least slow down its relentless progression. But, I liked that my aunt was re-living a joyful time in her life, stuck in anticipation of pleasure, and, despite Paul's giving me hell, I encouraged her: "I'm coming to the party, too," I would say. "Thanks for waiting for me."

I nod toward the Corridor Woman and pull myself forward past her by hand-over-hand gripping of the railing. I have never been good with machines "Push the right wheel forward," Colleen instructs me, "with your hand."

"Like this?" I am going to hit the wall.

"Push your left wheel backwards."

"Backwards?"

"Yes. That's how you can steer."

"Hi, Trevor," I say, as Colleen maneuvers me away from him. I am exhausted from thinking and pushing. I was a left-hander turned into a right-hander, and I never know what way to turn a wheel when backing up my car, and now I'm driving the damn wheelchair. I just don't know how things work.

"Is this the way out?" Trevor asks, pointing the wrong way.

"No." *At least I do know that!*

"Okay. Thanks."

I've reached the crossroads of the nation. Well, the crossroads of the Bellemont. And I am in a wheelchair traffic jam. Just behind me is the nursing station and Trevor. Straight ahead are the Administrative Offices and the Therapy Room. To the right is the dining room and to the left a corridor to the Family Room and the long-term wings. One balding woman is sitting in her wheelchair in the middle of the crossroads, a blank look on her face, but I think she likes being in the fray. Colleen pushes her wheelchair to the wall, and then pushes me the rest of the way to the Therapy Room, for which I will be eternally grateful.

My therapy today will begin on the NuStep. I consider the NuStep an extremely well-designed machine because even I can figure it out. Anyone who can sit in a recumbent bike position can use it. You can use one foot or two on the pedals, and one hand or two on the moveable handles. The resistance can be as low as "1" or as high as "10." You can be timed for one minute or thirty minutes. You can be as close to the pedals as "1" or as far as "16." I am an "11."

There are only two NuStep machines. Both are occupied. On one is a white-haired African American woman with strands of popbeads around her neck. She mumbles that people are not kind to her. She looks at me like she wants to spit on me. On the other NuStep is a man who has had a stroke. His thirty-something son is by his side, encouraging him. How difficult it must be for the son to see his father, who still looks trim and athletic in his Jack Nicholson golf shirt, weak and trembling with his left arm hanging useless by his side, left leg dangling to the floor. The son looks strong and handsome, an acorn off the old oak tree before him, an oak tree that is losing its limbs.

"You have to get off the NuStep now, Violet," Colleen says. "We have therapy clients now." Colleen helps Violet onto her wheelchair.

"I live here," Violet shouts. "I have rights. People aren't nice to me."

"She's a long-term resident," Colleen explains. "Not a rehab client. The long-timers can only use the machinery when we're not working with therapy clients. Violet's always wanting to be here."

I look through Violet's eyes. I wonder how I would feel if I were in the Bellemont long-term, but always a second-class citizen, always subject to displacement from the invasion and succession of temporary rehab clients.

"We'll try you for six minutes at level 3 today," Colleen says to me. She's all business. "How does that sound?" She winces.

"Like progress," I say. When I get on the NuStep, I see what Violet might love about the machine. It is positioned in front of picture windows. One can see the sky, trees, ground, and High Street, the comings and goings of trucks, cars, people. Sitting high-up on the NuStep is the only spot where a resident can see the natural and social worlds outside the Bellemont. Does Violet ever get to actually be in that world? And, what do the passersby see of the Bellemont? Clients working out? How nice.

"You've got a visitor," Colleen says to me, directing Celeste toward the NuStep. In the 1970s, we were in a women's support group together. The group encouraged her to follow her dream and become a minister. She officiated at my wedding to Ernest. Her first. She always has a smile for me.

"My husband dropped me off," she says. "He's waiting in the car. So I can't stay long."

"How wonderful of you to come," I say, as I work my NuStep.

"You look great, Laurel." Celeste has been privy to my frozen shoulders, tennis-elbow, and plantar fasciitis because we go to the same health club and are sometimes in the arthritic therapy pool at the same time.

"As we grow older," Celeste winks and smiles. "It's not one thing *after* another, it's one thing *on top* of another." She is ten years my senior. We laugh, and Celeste walks her walker on out.

My occupational therapist, Effie Lou, helps me off the NuStep back into my wheelchair, gives me my hand weights and an exercise cheat-sheet. Her pretty face looks haggard. I want to say "The blabbering substitute occupation therapist, Rhonda, told me you had some trouble at home yesterday," but instead I say, "Glad to have you back." I try to decide whether I can tell Effie Lou about my hallucinogenic experiences yesterday. For all I know, she may be required by law or professional ethics to report me to someone who will report me to someone who will put me in a psych ward for observation. I venture a non-self-disclosing question, "Do you know if Vicodin can have odd side effects?"

"My husban' Tony got a script for Vicodin for his back," she says. "He's bein' a little koo-ky."

"Thanks for pushing my chair," I say to Effie Lou as she wheels me down the hall.

"Ah need the ex-zer-cise," she says, her Kentucky accent in full force.

"Rhonda was just horrid," I say. I feel righteous, like a schoolgirl snitch. Effie Lou lets me tell the whole story of Rhonda being mean and putting me at risk. Effie Lou seems to enjoy my little rant. She assures me I won't have to work with Rhonda again.

"Hi, Trevor."
"Oh, Hi!"

"Come into my room," Renee says. She's in her doorway. "I've been waiting here for you." She adjusts her urine bag.
 "See you tomorrow," Effie Lou says.
Renee's room is smaller than mine and feels crowded. Her window faces the parking lot. Her bed is against the wall, facing toward the hall with a white curtain half-pulled around it. The air feels noxious, like it has gorged on sanitizing chemicals. On her table is a box of Kleenex, a glass of cranberry juice, a laptop, and a bouquet of silk flowers.
"I don't know if I am going to get through this, Laurel," Renee says.
I wait.
"They dropped me last night."
"Who did?"
"Like a football." Renee starts crying. She pulses her head, pokes it down.
"Who did?" I imagine Renee flailing on her back, powerless to get up, her pendulous breasts grazing the floor.
"Three of them. The mean one, the strong one and the ugly one."
 "Have you told the manager?" I ask.
"Yeah. I'm having X-rays taken of my shoulder."
"I'm so sorry, Renee."
"Why does everything bad happen to me?"

"Ready for a rest in your own bed, Laurel?" Brooke has come into Renee's room.
"Thanks," I say. I wave Renee a "high-five" good-bye.
Brooke wheels me into my room and helps me into my freshly made bed. A glass of cranberry juice is on my bedside table.

"Did you hear about Renee?" I ask.

Brooke nods.

"What happened?"

Brooke swallows some air, opens her eyes wide. She's deciding, I think, whether she can talk about another patient. She decides that she can. "Three staff were helping her in the bathroom, when she decided she could do it herself. She was covered with lotion and she slipped out of their hands and fell onto her back."

"I bet Vena was one of them."

Brooke doesn't deny it.

"And Kiendra?"

"Mmm…"

"And Jamal?"

"Ah…"

"I hope they don't fire Jamal. He's so new he's probably on probation."

"They won't fire him. They need him."

"They need a lot more aides than they have!"

"Call if you need me, Laurel. I'm going back to check on Renee."

I remember a radio interview with Sarah Sudoff, a photographer. The camera, she said, is like a flashlight, illuminating places of darkness, places we have overlooked or don't want to see—like medical procedures, hospitals, death. These are what she photographs. When asked if there was any photo she took that was too much, "too powerful, too raw," Sarah paused, as if contemplating whether it would be too much to talk about it. Then she did. A histology lab technician had told her they had just received an amputated leg. The person had diabetes, his leg was gangrous and amputating it saved his life. Did she want to see it? She did. The technician pulled the leg out on its cutting board. The fluorescent lights turned the cutting board bright green, the skin was moist, purple and red, with pieces of white bone sticking out. Sarah said, "It was stunningly beautiful, haunting and disturbing, this detached leg—"

I wonder how Renee would feel about having her "detached" leg ogled on its cutting board, shown to strangers, and photographed for a book called *Repositories.* I wonder how she would feel if she had heard this radio program. Outrage? Fear? Remorse that she hadn't seen her legs—how they looked "detached"?

Detached leg: In Tolstoy's *War and Peace,* the vain and handsome Prince Nikolai is wounded by a grenade that requires that his leg be amputated on the battle-field. "Show it to me!" He declares. "Show me my beautiful leg!" And the medics do.

I look down at my right leg's childhood leg wound, 47 stitches up my shin bone, and how ugly my leg looked, bone showing, flesh showing, blood. And then the ride in the paddy-wagon to the hospital with my older sister gloating that as "pretty" as I was, because of my wound I could never be a model when I grew up. I was five, she was fifteen.

"What? You have a scar on your leg?" Ernest asked me last year after reading a poem I had written about it.

And then I think about my mother, and how vain she was about her beautiful legs, and the mutual pleasure we had from me massaging her beautiful legs with lotion, her in a morphine twilight sleep, peacefully dying . And my sister's beautiful legs, endlessly restless, as she lay dying, in excruciating pain—her husband Paul controlling the morphine.

"Beauty is as beauty does," my father would caution. Then he'd sing a little Irish melody and blow me a kiss good-night.

Ring-ring.

"Hi, Ho-nee. "

"Hi, Ellyn." My friend Ellyn is a Kabalistic therapist who works in nursing homes in New Jersey. "How did you know to call just right now?"

"Telekinesis or sumthin' fancy like that." I imagine her chin pulled back, her bobbed white hair bobbing around her head.

I tell her about my hallucinations, and about my forty-five minutes of having to pee for before an aide came.

"I hear ya', Ho-nee," she says. "Needing to pee is the major complaint from my clients, too."

I find myself thinking about the job "nurses' aide." At the Bellemont, most of the aides are from Sierra Leone. A few are African Americans, and fewer are Anglo Americans. The aides are responsible for my feedings, bathing, dressing, toileting, bed linens, ambulatory assistance, taking vitals, light cleaning-up, and answering the call button. They have to deal with my changing moods, abruptness, and dogs. And I am one of the "better" patients.

"You shudda done what my clients do," Ellyn continues. "Pee in the bed. Or call 911. Or both."

Jingle-jangle.

"Lily! Bashi! I love you both!! Get on up here on my bed, the both of you!! *Really* be here now ... And you, too, Ernest ... I have a sorrowful story to tell you about Renee."

"Sunday dinner! Roast-beef , gravy and mashed potatoes." Brooke lifts the cover from the tray, wiggles her nose and says, "Smells good." Bashi and Lily are wiggling their noses, too, beside themselves with anticipation. Like all dog noses, their noses dominate their brains. They have about sixty times more scent-detecting cells than us odor-deprived humans. They also have a "smell memory bank." Each time they get a whiff of something they test it against the whiffs they've already had of stuff, judge it, categorize it, store it in their brains. Some dogs recognize 10,000 different smells. My Paps have had roast beef, gravy, and mashed potatoes before and lo! Here it is again. I signal Brooke to put the tray on the floor for the *real and alive* Papillons. A feast!

Linda M. and Brenda are at my door with a flourish of indigo-colored flowers in a translucent violet square vase. The colors match the clothes I have chosen to wear in rehab.

"See you in a little while," Ernest says. "Give you a chance to visit."

"How did you know those were my rehab colors?" I ask Linda.

"Thought they might be." Linda grins. She is my elfin friend, little, quick and bursting with life. "The colors of the Third-eye and Crown chakras." She is doing a little hip dance. "Indigo, it is said, gives you access to your subconscious awareness, letting you meet yourself with a new understanding. And violet—oh, Crown violet—the recognition that we are unfolding all the time—the expanded energy of simply Being—asking us to be here in this place and time. But you know all of that, don't you Laurel?"

Linda has a way of telling people new things in a way that makes them believe they already knew them. She's a living model of Platonic theory. She joined my postmodernist studies group about five years into its tenure. At first I was hesitant about the group inviting her because she was an administrator in my university, and I didn't know how that would affect our free-wheeling discussion. She did. But in a positive way, bringing in her spiritual zest for life.

"Okay, Dr. Linda, tell me about the square vase?" I know that the square symbolizes the four directions, but I am curious to hear her interpretation.

"Well, Dr. Laurel," Linda pulls herself up to her full five-foot stature and says, "It is a symbol for the earth. Grounding . . . Foundation . . . or," her spirits are bubbling out, "a symbol for the heart."

"Or for the four elements," her partner Brenda says. She looks like she could be the supermodel Iman's sister.

In 1970, I taught the first Women's Studies class at Ohio State University. Brenda was one of the hundred enrolled students. They ranged from freshmen to PhD level. We met once a week for four hours. There were no textbooks and precious little research, other than treating "sex" as a variable in statistical studies. I applied tenets from Women's Liberation to my teaching, such as making certain everyone had a chance to speak, in that period's vernacular, "to find her voice and speak her truth." Vastly different ideas were held by students, ideas they were passionate about. My teaching strategies (such as the "talking stick," small group discussions, topics proposed by students) rewarded civil exchange of the ideas in the classroom, and allowed me to teach sociological theory and research methods relevant to their study interests.

For me, teaching discussion classes is how I imagine I would perform as a courtroom defense lawyer. The same skill set, the same wiliness. First, you have to have your "facts" straight, know them, just like that, right off the top of your head, so the jury members (students) have confidence in your authority. Second, you have to listen carefully to the "testimonies" of "witnesses" (statements of students) so you can find the "contradictions" and "lead" them into their "truths." Third, you have to be to open to "surprise" witnesses (out-of-left-field ideas) and have strategies ready. Fourth, you have to make eye contact—smile, laugh—be likeable, so the jury (students) will listen to your summaries—find your client innocent (learn and do well on their exams.) And fourth, if all goes well—well, you go home feeling great.

This is not just idle speculation. A mixed-methods research project conducted by Anne Statham, Judith Cook, and myself on gender and university teaching found that for women to receive positive student evaluations, they had to be judged as both competent and likeable. Men only had to appear competent; if they were liked, their ratings went sky-high. Women professors felt good when a class went well, depressed when it did not. Male professors felt good when they learned something new. These same results have held true for trial attorneys. They probably hold true for all the professions requiring social interaction where there is a power/knowledge imbalance—like doctors over patients.

Word spread that the Sociology of Women class was the place to be. Students added the course. They were sitting on the floor and on the windowsills. Soon, there was standing room only. Extra sessions were added to accommodate panels of visitors on different issues such as sexuality, occupations, relationships, pop culture, and religion. One panel on Reproductive Rights: Choice vs. Pro-Life brought speakers from the pro-life organization's headquarters in Cincinnati. At the close of the panel, these visitors refused to stop talking, to stop accusing women of being murderers, and refused to leave. I called the campus police, who escorted them out of my classroom. They filed a complaint with my department chair. He defended me and the course.

This first Sociology of Women class was the most creatively and intellectually stimulating class I have ever taught. Not only did I hone my lawyerly skills, I used my modeling and theatrical ones. I created and acted characters—like Pugilistic Sperm and Passive Ovum. The clothes I chose to wear matched the topic, as if the classroom were a runway or a proscenium. On days that the class was given over to student presentations, I wore only unobtrusive black clothing, like a scene-changer might wear.

My textbook on gender grew out of the teaching. Many students have told me that the class changed their lives by giving them not just permission but reason and fodder to follow their career and relationship dreams. Brenda was one of those students.

"Well, just look at those sweet Papillons," Linda M. says. She and Brenda have two large German Shepherd-mix dogs. I think each one weighs more than Linda, and that Brenda must be the disciplinarian.

"I love these Paps," Brenda says. "Can they have a treat?"

I nod.

"Brenda's a complete pushover for any dog," Linda says. "She likes to spoil them. I like to train them."

Linda picks up Lily and Brenda picks up Bashi. They massage their backs in a zigzag manner that I remember reading about as soothing to dogs.

We three humans begin a lengthy conversation about dogs.

About two years ago, I woke up and said to Ernest that I didn't know why but I wanted a little dog. We have two cats—we always have had cats—so wanting a dog seemed odd, but true. I started reading dog books, watching dog programs, and researching dog breeds online. I wanted everything from my dog: beauty, agility, sweetness, smarts. Papillons met my criteria. My dog-loving friend Pat set us up with Liselle, a show-dog breeder from Indiana. She brought two 15-month-olds to meet us in a pet store near Dayton. The female was tiny, lithe and unusual in her brindle-coloredness; the male was swaggery, yappy, and typically patterned, black and white. We sat on chairs and Ernest put the female on his lap. "That's the one," I said to Liselle. "We'll take her." Then the male jumped into my lap, put his head on my forearm, and looked up at me with winsomeness. "He's chosen you," Ernest said. Ernest and I conferred. "We'll take both of them," we said.

"Thought you might," Liselle said. "That's good. Papillons like having another Papillon as a housemate." We've only had Lily and Bashi as our housemates for a year, but we cannot imagine life without them.

"People are always asking me why I have dogs at this time in my life," I say. "Ernest says just tell them 'We don't know why, yet.'"

"They bring us happiness and comfort," Brenda says. "Something outside of ourselves to take care of."

"They connect our human souls to other species' souls," Linda says.

I ponder that and think for a bit about women who run with the wolves.

"Isn't it interesting that all dog breeds evolved from the wolf?" I say.

"Women did the domesticating," Brenda says, "by choosing not to cook the more docile camp-following wolf pups."

"We bred them for special purposes, too—like catching rats or encircling dangerous prey," adds Linda.

"Taking them with us as we migrated," I say. "Wherever we are, dogs are."

"Some ethnologists believe that humans could not have survived without the help of dogs; that our two species are symbiotic." Linda is glowing. "Isn't that a wonderful magical mystery?"

"See you later, Lily." Linda gives her a final massage and sets her down.

"Good boy, Bashi," Brenda says, surreptitiously giving Bashi another little treat.

I have known these two women for over forty years, and this is the first time I have spent time alone with the two of them. I didn't realize until now that we shared so much more than our histories as academics.

"Hi, Jean," I say. Her black hair is cut into a bob. She leaves her North Face ski jacket on.

"Thanks for coming," I say.

"I like your bed jacket."

"A friend lent it to me," I say. "So I could look dressed up."

Jean is a close friend, a member of my Art League. We have lunch every couple of weeks and talk about our artwork. We have been emailing almost daily for the past two years, ever since Jean's lymphoma returned. I know it is very hard for her to come to the nursing home, to see the terminally sick people here. Our conversation is awkward, strained.

"Should I email you?" Jean asks.

"I'm not sure if the WiFi is working here," I say.

"Then, I'll phone you every day."

"Is everything okay?" The business manager, Brandon, is at the door.

"Is the WiFi working?" I ask. I haven't tried to access my email yet. It is freeing, not being wired-up. I like my do-nothing, moments of resting, and then resting again. It is lovely. Surely, there is nothing on my email that matters.

"I'll get the password from my boss," he says. "Tomorrow."

"Mark?" I am surprised by how happy I am to see him. He is the senior minister at Columbus's First Unitarian-Universalist Church of which I am a friend.

"How're you doing, Laurel?" He gives me a little hug. He is a little overweight and pale. "Your being in here was announced in church this morning."

"I really want to talk to you," I say, surprising myself even more. What do I want to talk about?

"Hi, Mom." I hear my younger son Josh's distinctive voice, soft, yet certain, and can smell his distinctive scent of organic cigarette tobacco.

"Hi, Grandma." Josh's son, Akiva. His voice, fast and crackly. The two saunter into my room and give me hugs.

I introduce Josh and Akiva. "Mark, meet Josh. He was in Sunday school at First UU before you became its minister."

"Yeah. I liked climbing the trees. Outside."

"And meet my grandson, Akiva. He went to the Church's pre-school."

"Happy to meet you," Akiva says, shaking Mark's hand and looking him straight in the eye.

"This is your family time," Mark says. "I can come back on—say—Wednesday afternoon."

"Sounds great!"

Josh sits on a chair at the foot of my bed. He is six-foot-six and maybe weighs 170 pounds. He looks like my father, sandy-red hair and large brown eyes. He doesn't take off his pea coat. Akiva sits down next to him. He is seventeen, six-foot-two, eyes of blue, and reddish-brown ringlets that reach past his shoulders. He looks like Michelangelo's *David*. He is not wearing a jacket. He takes off his sandals and cracks his knuckles.

"Sorry, I haven't gotten here sooner, Mom," Josh says. "I've had a load of homework. Math homework is insane." When Josh turned 18, a month before high-school graduation, he marched into the principal's office and dropped out of school. Then he came home, told me what he had done, packed his gear and moved to Cincinnati, where he became a busboy in a Chinese restaurant. My pain was immense—not only because he had dropped out of school, but because of the assumptive question asked by friends, colleagues and family: "So where is Josh going to college?" He wasn't. I felt guilt and shame. My failure as mother was apparent. That year was one of the saddest years in my life.

Josh did move back to Columbus to live with his father, Herb. He began a career as a leathersmith and furniture maker. To make money he became a master mechanic. After hurting his back at the BMW dealership, he could no longer work on cars or construct furniture. He gave in. He enrolled in college with three majors—math, bio-math, and molecular engineering. This year he is a senior.

"How are you feeling, Grandma?" Akiva asks.

"Not bad," I say. Akiva is my only biological grandchild. I have a deep affinity with him, not because he is my biological grandchild, but because I can see "*me*" in him—in his quirkiness, quickness, and appetites. We both detest coconut and beets and clothing tags that scratch at the neck.

Akiva has been home-schooled most of his life. Last year, his mother, Suzanne, enrolled him in an online high school. Akiva rebelled, dropped out, and moved to his dad's house. He is not talking to his mother and doesn't plan to until he is his "own person." He has been living with Josh for a year, now. Plans are that he take his GED exam and matriculate at the community college.

"Suzanne was here yesterday," I say. "She helped me a lot with my wheelchair."

"She's had a lot of experience with wheelchairs," Akiva says.

"Did she say when she was getting remarried?" Josh asks.

"No . . . I think she's waiting for . . . "

"She knows I will come to the wedding," Akiva says. "That's important."

"Glad to hear that," I say.

Akiva plays air-cello.

"So, how's the cello coming, Akiva?" I ask.

"Good. I'm back to my old teacher."

Five years ago, I bought Akiva a student cello. He rapidly progressed through chamber strings, quartets, and cadet orchestra until, at fifteen, he refused to audition for the symphony's youth orchestra. "It isn't fun," he said. "Everyone is too serious. Tiger-moms!" For the next two years, although he took expensive lessons with a "tiger-teacher," he practiced less and less. "I don't want to be around musicians," he ranted. "They're always in their heads listening to music. They don't listen to you when you're talking to them. There are more things in life than music."

My heart churned over this turn of events. Music was one of the strings that tied us together. We had similar tastes—Bach, Vivaldi, and the Moody Blues. His piano teacher, a retired music professor, believed that Akiva could concertize in piano or cello or both. "Shall I refer you to my alma mater, Yale Music School?" he had asked. Akiva declined. I can't imagine what else Akiva could do with his life.

"So, how's the League of Legends game?" I ask.

"Good."

"Latin?"

"Good."

"Faux-Pas-The-Cat?"

"Good."

"Seen any good movies lately?"

Akiva puts on his sandals, looks at his dad.

"We've not had time," Josh says. "I'm sorry we have to go, Mom. I've got a big test tomorrow and Akiva's friend Zach is coming over."

They lean over to hug me.

"We'll be back on Thursday after Akiva's cello lesson, and on Sunday, again."

"That'll be nice."

CHECK HALL 100 EXIT CHECK HALL 100 EXIT CHECK HALL 100 EXIT RRRRRRRRIIIIINNNNNNGGGGGG RRRRRRRRIIIIINNNNNNGGGGGG

"Is that your family just left?" Renee asks, wheeling towards my door.

Renee people-watches outside her door as if our rehab corridor is Central Park.

"My son and grandson," I say.

"The one with the long hair?"

"My seventeen year-old grandson."

"He's hot."

CHAPTER 3

"Help Me ... Help Me"

January 9

I have an understanding of my days. The morning routines, the afternoon and evening visits from family, friends, staff, dogs, and my neighbor Renee, punctuated with periods of quiet, rest, and rumination. The shape of my time stays pretty much the same, but the players in it change. There is something reassuring in this. All my needs for food, water, and care are met—if not at once, eventually. I am never bored. And I can close my door, close out the din, the grunts, the calls for help.

This morning Brooke has fixed my Rice Chex and rice milk with raisins and bananas she hijacked from the kitchen. She has helped me with a sponge bath, found a pair of wide-legged pajama bottoms and encouraged me to see if they can fit over my wrapped up foot, which they can. She finds my violet top in the closet and my new purple velour hoodie. I get dressed for the first time in five days. I feel better. Less sick. Less scared. Less less.

"I have the password for the computer, now," Brandon says. He is wearing a different blue shirt and tie set today. He takes my laptop and enters the code. "It doesn't seem to be working. I'll find another one," he says with embarrassment.

"All set for therapy," Colleen sidles into my room. She cringes as she wheels me into the corridor. Just like the apocryphal cobbler's son who doesn't have the shoes he needs, my p.t. doesn't have the p.t. she needs. Can't another p.t. help her? Maybe she needs more than they can do for her ... I hope she doesn't fall ...

Renee is not in the hallway and her door is closed. Trevor is in his usual place, the nurses in theirs, and soon I am in mine on the NuStep, now set for ten minutes at resistance level 4. I can see Rhonda-the-Horrid working over an older woman who is on oxygen. "Check her blood-oxygen level," Colleen shouts to Rhonda. The poor old woman is as white and sticky-looking as leftover rice. The long-term resident Violet is on the other NuStep wearing a different collection of pop bead necklaces. An electric wheelchair is in the room with a large card attached to its basket—*Happy Anniversary Violet!* "Time to get off the NuStep," Colleen says to her. "I'll help you into your brand new electric wheelchair!" Violet sneers down her nose at me. Effie Lou works me on my hand weights and pushes me into the hallway.

"So how's it going at home?" I ask.

"Ah'm thinking 'bout takin' a diff'rent job as a home-health occupational therapist. It'll pay a lot more and I kin set my hours." Effie Lou says.

"How come?"

"Tony's son A. J. probly goin' have to come live by us. His muthah is a druggie and she's neglectin' A. J. He's thirteen. Boys can git into big trouble."

"How often does Tony see A. J. now?"

"Ev'ry other week-end."

"How does A. J. feel about you?"

"He calls me some names Ahm not gonna repeat."

We pass by the nurses, Trevor, and the grunting Corridor Woman. Renee's door is still closed.

"You're all dressed up today," Effie Lou pauses. "Ah bet you'd like your hair warshed, and Mildred's here. She comes on Mondays and Tuesdays. Your first warsh is free."

I nod my approval and Effie Lou wheels me past my door and into the wing of the long-term residents. Doors are open. The rooms have two beds. I hear and see the "Help me . . . help me" man stretched on his bed on his back, and I see his roommate, stretched on his back, rhythmically moaning. The corridor's width is narrowed by residents in wheelchairs on both sides. They are dressed with no place to go. An actress friend said that seeing one person in a wheelchair was tragic, but seeing a line of them was comedy. I see nothing funny here.

Effie Lou wheels me to the end of the hall. On the left is the Activities Room, and on the right, the Beauty Shop. Two women's heads are under old-fashioned dryers, a third is having a perm. All three have blank stares. Tattered hair-style magazines are on the windowsill. The television is blaring. No one is watching. The Beauty Shop is a spot of faux normalcy. It looks like the kind of shop the Bellemont residents probably frequented, neighborhood shops like "Marjory's Cut and Curl" or "Patsy's Curl and Cut" before the Midwestern hair-styling industry was upscaled into salons and spas and franchised by beauty-product manufacturers. I hope the vacant-eyed customers feel good here at Mildred's, or if not, that their families, who are probably footing the bill, think they do.

"Mildred, this is Laurel," Effie Lou says. "She wants her hair warshed."

"Hi, Laurel," Mildred says. She looks like an elderly Lucille Ball.

I imagine that Mildred once was chief proprietor of "Mildred's Shampoo and Set" on High Street in lower Clintonville, but her independent small business became increasingly iffy as she and her clientele aged, and younger customers wanted jaggety cuts and ombre-colored hair shaded like a gradient from dark at the roots to sun-kissed at the tips. She did not embrace the new aesthetic. Rather than retire, she rented spaces in nursing homes, to the benefit of all, it would seem. Women always want their hair done.

My mother went every week to the beauty shop to get her thick black hair washed and set. She always looked well-coifed. As she lay in her bed dying, her silver and gray hair spread over the pillow. "I didn't know you had your hair colored and roots touched up," I said. "Ssh," she said. "Father doesn't know." When I had my long hair cut in Sassoon's in New York City and came out looking like a refugee from Russia, my then six-year-old son, Ben, said, "I know why they call it a beauty shop. They take away your beauty."

"I can be with you in about twenty-minutes," Mildred says. "Can you wait? Or do you want to come back tomorrow? The other days I am at other homes."

"I'll wait in the Activities Room," I say. "I'll do my email. I think I saw a computer there."

"Oh, do you know how to do email?" Mildred asks. My approval rating has gone up. "They just got the computer. They're offering lessons once a week. I might take them, too."

I manage to wheel myself over to the Activities Room. The Director is at her desk. She nods at me and continues her paper work, cutting out black shapes for the Friday-the-Thirteenth party, I think.

"I need some help turning on the computer," I say to the Director.

"Push the power button."

"I can't find it."

"It's . . . oh well . . ." She gets up from her desk, walks the twelve feet to the computer, pushes a master-button on the floor and the computer wakes-up. "I guess you wouldn't be able to reach it from your wheelchair."

"Thanks," I say, wondering if the master-button had been purposely placed to prevent the residents, most of whom are in wheelchairs, from free access to the computer—or just mindlessly placed. I do my trillion emails by deleting the most of them, saving those that require an answer until I can do so at my leisure in my own room. I turn my attention to the books.

When I was in graduate school, I arranged my books by color. There weren't many of them. In my house, now, although I have given over seventy boxes of books to public and university libraries, I am surrounded by books—almost overwhelmed, oppressed. In the basement there are perhaps seventy feet of bookshelves that Ernest designed and made. On one shelf are journals that contain an article that I've written; on another are novels-I-like, arranged alphabetically by author; on a third are travel books, arranged geographically from East to West; fourth and fifth shelves house a complete set of black-leatherette

Agatha Christie mysteries (including her unreadable autobiography), a set Ernest and I bought one book at a time, twenty years ago, thinking we'd read them (again) when we retired (which we have, but haven't); a shelf of my childrens' books that still mean something to me, although apparently not to the children or grandchildren as they haven't taken them; and a diminished shelf of sociology and psychology books, arranged by color. I still own my graduate school tomes.

I like thinking about my home and my books. I miss them.

In my living room, there are three bookcases. One holds books written by Ernest or me. He went on a book tour for one of his novels, *Prince Elmo's Fire,* as did I for one of my sociology books, *The New Other Woman.* Book tours are not fun or glamorous. Much of the time you are waiting for an airplane or a carry-out lunch or you are in the Green Room of a television program whose host may decide not to interview you, or you're in a radio studio fielding phone calls from the Angry or the Hurt and you are telling everything about your book and nobody who is listening is going to buy it anyway, or you are in a bookstore with piles of your book on a table in front of you and nobody has come. Your publisher has told you to sign every book because then they can't be returned. How many remaindered books have I left behind me? I feel guilty thinking about that.

Book tours are pretty much over with now. Newspapers have cut their book review sections, radio stations have dumped their author interviews—unless the authors are celebrities or connected to the station, and television promotes—well, television. Independent bookstores (like independent beauty shops) have shut their doors. With Nook, Kindle, and iPads, who needs brick and mortar? Everything I read about the publishing industry repeats the same thing: We just don't know the future.

Thinking about book publishing is exhausting...I need to return to my home, my book shelves.

On three shelves on the living room's first bookcase there are thirty-five years of photograph albums: our wedding, and travels to Europe, Russia, the Middle-East, Australia, the Caribbean, Mexico, Bermuda, near every direction in the United States, and birthdays, holidays, family visits . . . Several empty place-holding albums and a overflowing box of unfiled photos . . . and now the realization that pictures from the last few years are not printed, but on discs and flash drives. Have homey personal photo albums gone the way of book stores? Gone into an electronic netherland?

The second bookcase holds books by friends and family, art books, and pretty things, too, like antique Russian boxes, glass sculptures, and two silver goblets. The third case holds poetry, anthologies first, and the rest arranged alphabetically. This is the only bookcase in which the books Ernest and I each brought to the marriage are nestled spine-to-spine.

I like thinking about books . . .

I like acquiring books. If I am interested in a topic, I want to have a mini-library about it. When I am through with the topic, I like to give them to good homes. This year I gave away my mini-library on the Holocaust to Congregation Beth Tikvah, my mini-library on feminist spirituality to Jung House, and my mini-library on post-modernist themes to a struggling graduate student. Other mini-libraries are still in my study: books on book-making, art books, architecture, dreams, writing—and a new one—dogs. Each little library is separated from the others, and each is arranged alphabetically.

On a shelf in my study are some books that represent my spiritual journeying. On one end of that shelf is the only book of mine my mother kept after I left home. It is called, *A Little Lower than the Angels.* It was the workbook that accompanied my confirmation class at Anshe Emet Synagogue in Chicago. It was all about science, morality, and Jews as an evolving culture. A theology without a God. I had written on the cover in indelible ink: IF LOST DO NOT RETURN. Next to it are the *I Ching, Encyclopedia of Goddesses, Good News Bible, Emerson Essays,* theodicy books, *Heal Yourself, Courage to Change,* and the five books of Moses in English and Hebrew. At the other end of the shelf is *The Zohar* (radiance), the foundation of the Jewish mystical thought, Kabala. I don't pretend to understand the book but I am intrigued and comforted by its vision. Human-beings are said to have sparks of the Divine within them. Unlike angels, who are like plants, standing still and getting taller, humans can walk around and make radical shifts. We rank higher than the angels.

So many books to think about…

We learn so much about others by perusing their book shelves, a sanctioned nosiness that I cannot resist when left alone, or not, in a room that has books on shelves. As if I am a field anthropologist, I note genre, authors, content, new or used looking, paper or hard back. And, then, too, I can learn something I didn't know about the owner's world-view because asking about what someone thinks and feels about a particular book is acceptable social interaction, neither intrusive or inappropriate as it might be if I asked, for example, about bills or prescription bottles on a table or socks under a couch. Non-intrusive methods of discovery I think are the finest.

What am I learning about myself as I peruse my own shelves?

In my studio are books I've not yet made. Beautiful Japanese and French papers for covers, hand-made text-blocks, cover boards, acid-free glue. These unmade books do not oppress me. I like potentiality.

… thinking about the books inside my house puts me into my house…

On the upstairs bookshelves are the books I love: books I have made by hand and dog-eared, collectable children's books, surrounded by child-size tea sets, little dolls that remind me of my childhood, and sewing boxes that belonged to my mother. My sons know that these are the books and objects that have mattered to me, and might matter to them. I arranged those shelves before my ankle surgery . . . Just in case I did die . . .

Now, thinking about how one might arrange books amuses me. I remember teaching about how Victorians separated male and female authors for propriety's sake, and how the Dewey Decimal system reflected cultural desires for efficiency—everything having a proper place, everything in its proper place. And then came the Library of Congress system preferred by universities and, well, Congress. Its indented system is much like an outline in which all knowledge is divided into twenty-one basic categories, each identified by a single letter of the alphabet and then off we go into an alpha-numerical maze through which books the library already owns are identified. But here, in the Bellemont's library, there is no discernible order. Prettier books have been put on a credenza, paperbacks on a cart. There are fewer books here than on any one of my bookshelves at home. I browse and find two books about dogs and wonder-of-all-wonders, *Seven Centuries of Verse,* red and scuffed looking, just like the one I used in my undergraduate humanities classes. I clutch the three books to my dressed-up bosom.

"Ready for your hair wash?" Mildred asks. "I'll wheel you back to your room afterwards."

"Thanks," I say as Mildred helps me into my bed. I feel taken care of, the way I did when I was a young girl with hair halfway down my back. I would stand on an apple crate in front of the large kitchen sink and my ten-year older sister, Jessica, would lather me up, scratch my scalp, run her fingers through my hair as she rinsed it with water, neither too hot nor too cold, neither too hammery nor too wimpy, but just right. She Turkish-toweled my hair, brushed and braided it. She was grooming me, the way our primate relatives do their kin. She was showering me with visceral love. No wonder I grew up to love her dearly.

"Well, this is a wonderful surprise," I say, seeing my new Artist Way friend Nancy coming into my room. She is managing her cane well. She has the sweetest smile and voice. Last autumn, she had right knee replacement surgery and rehabbed at Gahanna Center. On the day before she was to leave for home, she reached for a light-switch in her bathroom. Her wheelchair flew out from beneath her. She could hear her left ankle bones break as she hit the wall. The right knee replacement split open. She lay on the bathroom floor for a quarter hour before someone came. After her fall, her knee replacement had to be replaced and six bolts were needed to hold her ankle in place. She was transferred to the rehab wing at the Bellemont where she lay in bed for over three weeks, unable to put weight on either leg. Then, because she was not "progressing," the rules required she be moved to the unskilled nursing wing. I wonder how often she had to call 911 in that wing.

Nancy puts a vase of yellow roses on my table.

"Well, look who's here!" Brooke has floated in. She gives Nancy a big hug. "You look wonderful. It is wonderful to see you again."

"You've given me hope," I say to Nancy. "Hope and roses."

Nancy gives me a little kiss on my cheek and gets ready to leave.

"Let me wheel you out, Laurel," Brooke says. "We'll try to keep up with Nancy."

Renee's door is ajar and I can hear her weeping as Brooke pushes my wheelchair into my corridor toward the exit door. I wave good-by to Nancy.

Jingle-jangle.

"You look spiffy today, Darlin," Ernest says, kissing me on the cheek. "I can wheel her back," he tells Brooke.

"Yap."

"Yap."

"Is that Lily?" Renee's in the corridor.

"Yap."

"Yap."

"Come here, Lily," Renee says. She has a bruise on her cheek and is holding her left arm akimbo.

Ernest puts Lily on Renee's lap. Her thighs bounce forward. Bashi looks anxiously at me.

"Do you want to sell Lily? How much would she cost? I'll have lots of money once my lawyer settles my claim against the doctor who did this to me," she says pointing to her absent legs. "And even more once I sue this place for dropping me and hurting my shoulder."

"Not for sale, Renee," Ernest says, gently taking Lily off Renee's lap. He opens my door and wheels me into my spiffed-up room. A new bouquet of flowers has arrived. It has the scent of spring. The card says, "Be Well, Love, Brenda and Linda M."

"Happiness is two warm, furry bodies on my bed," I say, "And flowers from friends and a poetry book."

"Books are going the way of the di-no-saur," Ernest says in his exaggerated Hoosier accent, letting the accent simultaneously give authority to the assertion and undercut it.

I think about my friend Marilyn. She is a retired English professor, five years older than I. She has been a beacon for me for forty years. She is the only person I know that I consider a role model. Last year, she reduced her private library to one shelf, keeping but one book from each of her favorite authors. Is that what I'll do when I get home? Depopulate my shelves, extinguish the lot of them.

"Books as endangered species?" I ask Ernest.

"Yep. Good idea. I think I'll cut my book-herd again." Like me, Ernest has given many boxes of books to the university. Recently he has sent family books to the Ross Lockridge, Jr. collection at the Lily Library in Bloomington. The towering bookshelves in his study, though, still hold Hemingway, Faulkner, Fitzgerald, Henry James, Thomas Wolfe, Kingsley Amis, and other "minor" writers.

"I don't think you're ready to let any of them go," I say.

Ernest takes his Kindle out of his pocket. "I could fit them all in here."

"Outside a dog, a book is a person's best friend," I say.

"Inside a dog, it's too dark to read," Ernest completes our favorite Groucho Marx quip.

"Hello, Laurel." The business-manager Brandon is at the door. I introduce him to Ernest and the dogs. Brandon nods his hello. "I've got a different code for your computer, now. It should work. The router is in the room next to you." He takes my laptop and encodes it. "You're on the internet now. I'll set it for Google."

"I heard you were here." My Art League friend Randy's high-pitched voice. He peeks in.

"Come in, Randy," I say. He gives Ernest a hug.

"Oh look!" He notices Bashi. "Tickle-tickle... You are so handsome... tickle-tickle." He rubs Bashi behind his ears. Bashi wags his tail. Randy's hair is black and white like Bashi's fur. "My older sister's in the long-term wing... Room 2060," Randy says. "Here, I'll write it down for you. I'll put it here so you won't lose it." He picks up my daybook and pens the room number on the fly-sheet. "I'm bringing my sister some romance novels... She likes to read them... She can't do much else... totally bedridden... crossword puzzles, she likes, too... I've brought her some of those, too... and some butterscotch lozenges, she likes, too....She's been here for eight months... Her money is running out... You could visit her... Room 2060... I'll be back next week, and I'll bring my two Chihuahuas... Sorry, I have to go now."

Ernest is settled into his chair by the window. He's Kindle-ing a biography of James Dickey. We met James Dickey perhaps twenty-five years ago. He had come to the University with his young, beautiful, healthy-looking, strong wife who turned out to be a heroin addict. Dickey was supposedly "on the wagon," but at the cubed-cheese and cheap red wine reception that followed his reading he gulped down a glass or three.

"Do you remember what Dickey read when we met him?" I ask Ernest. I am feeling sentimental, on the edge of melancholy, as my thoughts move from inanimate books to colorful memories.

"For his finale, he read a rhyming children's poem," Ernest says.

"Dickey would read a line and then have the audience shout out the next line's rhyming word—like call and ball, or choke and bloke. It was quite interactive, highly unusual for a poetry reading. Highly unusual for Dickey, too, who eschewed rhyme—loved rhythm and odd meters." Ernest pauses. He is just getting started. Ask him a literary question—well, any question—and he is a storehouse of information. "I think his signature theme was juxtaposing nature against civilization, the rawness and violence of nature against the suppression of culture."

I am thinking to myself, What would James Dickey have to say about the Bellemont? About any nursing home? Here I experience the primitive sensations and impulses associated with nature, and I hear the moans and weeping of the creatures in other dens; life's carnage kept alive through the intervention of civilization's needles, pacemakers, aspirators.

Like others of his generation of poets and philosophers, Dickey accepted the idea of dualism. Everything could be divided into two different, often warring parts, like good vs. bad, alive vs. dead, rational vs. emotional, male vs. female, and, Dickey's pet, nature vs. culture. The list is endless—fact vs. fiction, prose vs. poetry and that which I cut my academic teeth on: science vs. humanities.

A book that enthralled my graduate school professors was C. P. Snow's *The Two Cultures and the Scientific Revolution.* Snow argued that scientists were illiterate in the humanities, and that humanists were illiterate in science. Not knowing the second law of thermodynamics, Snow said, was equivalent to not knowing who Shakespeare was; not being able to define mass or acceleration was equivalent to not being able to read. If sociology were to bridge the two cultures it would have to be literate in both of them. The first question on my PhD oral examination was, "Apply the second law of thermodynamics to sociology."

The idea of a divide between the sciences and humanities was particularly trenchant for sociology. Departments determined, I think, to get a good share of governmental cold war largesse, beefed up claims to be a *science.* Statistics classes became the backbone of a sociological education. I was even enlisted to teach them, although I had never taken one, because I was "good at math"; my dissertation topic was a study of pure mathematics and I was then married to a mathematician.

Research methods seminars taught *scientific* methods of sampling and surveying populations to test deductively constructed hypotheses. Long established methods such as interviewing and participant-observation were rejected as *subjective* or seen as a kind of *foreplay* to the main research event, climaxing in an article in a top-ranked journal, and then the opportunity to snag another grant. And so, a new and pernicious division within sociology was reified: quantitative vs. qualitative. Snow's main point was missed: to solve problems, the two cultures *need* each other. Some researchers try to do this through *mixed methods*, reaching into quantitative and qualitative *toolboxes* (note not cosmetics bags). I have done that myself. But, over the past few decades the philosophical underpinning of the "two cultures" has been discredited. Bye-bye, bifurcation.

"You see, Mr. Dickey," I imagine he and I are having high tea, "Duality has bit the dust."

Mr. Dickey slathers his scone.

"*Doubt* that anyone has cornered the *Truth*," I trot out the first clause of my oft given lecture on postmodernism.

"I get it," he says. "Scientists once thought light was either a wave or a particle. But now they think it is both depending on how it is studied. And tomorrow, they'll think something different."

I move quickly down the lecture notes in my brain and say, "Boundaries between literary genre..."

"What boundaries?" He takes a bite of his scone. "Practicing novelists knows that they don't make it all up. The idea that there is *fiction* is a Fiction!" He slurps his tea.

"Well, and yes," I barge on. "All writing depends upon literary techniques—particular tropes that signal to readers how they are supposed to take in what they are reading."

He shrugs. Takes another scone bite.

"Bending," I assert.

"Gender," he answers.

I decide to veer from my canned lecture. "Mr. Dickey, I have a story to tell you."

He puts down his teacup.

"Last autumn, I signed up for a class at the community center. The registration form gave me three choices for my gender: Male, Female, Undecided."

"Undecided…hmm…" Mr. Dickey's nose wiggles while he's thinking. "That's how it is for most everything, now, huh…hmm…undecided…the big and small questions…When does life begin?…When does life end? What is life?"

"And that brings us, Mr. Dickey, to the division between nature and culture that you have extolled."

He nods his head.

"We're all cyborgs, Mr. Dickey—or will be, if we use modern medicine for restorative or enhancement purposes." I blink my eyes. I've had cataract surgery and the artificial lenses have enhanced my vision by correcting my astigmatism and myopia. Friends have had hip and knee replacements, prosthetic legs, and cochlear and pacemaker implants. Medical advances have produced nerve-grafting techniques that let a person operate a fully robotic limb. Electrodes planted in the brain of paralyzed people let them communicate to an external computer to power their wheelchairs. Implanted chips in eyes are restoring sight and a similar process for the vocal cords is restoring voice. Artificial hearts are beating.

"Not just human cyborgs either, Mr. Dickey," I say. "My dogs have GPS chips. So do my cats. The military is developing cyborg insects to fly over and detect explosives. Scientists have created remote-controlled beetles and lift-assisted moths. Pigeons are next."

"So, will we be able to choose to enhance ourselves?" Mr. Dickey looks sly.

"The transhumanists want that," I say. "They believe that the new technologies will help humans resist disease and aging and improve one's speed, intelligence, strength and the like…Kind of like getting upgrades until we are *posthuman*."

Mr. Dickey pushes back his chair.

"Given the spiraling out-of-control health costs for just restorative medicine, I cannot imagine funding for the transhumanist medical agenda, *my body, my choice*—voluntary organ replacements, brain, eye and ear implants and voluntary amputations, because prosthetics are better." I take a breath. "Nor do I think it should be funded. The values that propel the movement are robotic ones—efficiency and functionality—not the humanist ones." I am feeling nauseated. I need to think more about all of this... all around me in the Bellemont is suffering. Could it be prevented? Can it be ameliorated? And look at me... I had the financial wherewithal to pay for better lenses to enhance my eyesight... so I did... And what is underlying all of this? I am not sure how to think about it all... later... later....

"I wish my eye-sight had been better. I'd go for an eye-chip," Mr. Dickey says, getting up and ambling out the door.

"Boy!" Ernest's expletive brings me out of my ponderings. "Dickey lied about being a World War II night-flight pilot. He failed the eyesight test."

"Huh? Why are you telling me that now?" I ask

"I just read it. Boy, that shatters his mystique."

It is not that unusual for Ernest and me to be thinking the same things at the same time, whether awake or asleep, near each other or miles apart, communicating by email. For awhile I kept a dream journal in which I recorded our shared or overlapping dreams. I stopped doing that when it seemed no longer surprising.

Now, Ernest begins to read out loud to me about James Dickey's life. I close my eyes and "go" into the words, the way I "go" into music. How many years has it been since Ernest has read to me? Being read to is one of life's great blessings... *A human-to-human blessing...*

"Are you falling asleep?" he asks. "Shall I stop?"

"No and no. I love it."

"Hi Laurel," Jamal says. "Did I wake you? Okay if I take your vitals?"

"So, what happened that Renee got dropped like a football?"

"She wouldn't let us help her in the bathroom. She fought us, and she had lotion on, and…she slipped…I was against the wall…I wasn't touching her…She fell…"

"Is she badly hurt?"

"They've been taking X-rays today."

Jamal pats the dogs, straightens my coverlet, and points to *Seven Centuries of Verse.*

"Do you like poetry?" Ernest asks.

"I do," Jamal says, looking toward the floor. "Call if you need me, Laurel."

So many things gone—beauty parlors, book stores, printed photographs…Humans next?

I open *Seven Centuries of Verse* as if it is the I-Ching. Page 271, *Auguries of Innocence* by William Blake (1757–1827):

> To see a World in a Grain of Sand
> And a Heaven in a Wild Flower,
> Hold Infinity in the Palm of your Hand,
> And Eternity in an Hour.

CHAPTER 4

What Is Right

January 10

"Good Morning, Laurel." Jamal's voice.

"Hi. You're working double-shift, Jamal? Where's Brooke?"

"Brooke had a family emergency." Jamal paces around my room, as if he has something on his mind that's he not ready to let off his mind. He looks at my books and picks up the novel *Colonel Pettigrew's Last Stand.* "Was this good?"

"It was. It's funny and sad. Would you like to borrow it?"

He nods yes, and paces around some more. The request for the novel, I think, is all he is ready to say. I let it go.

"Hi Laurel." Brandon-the-business-manager has come in. "How'd the internet work?"

"It didn't," I say. "Access to WiFi was one of the questions I asked before agreeing on this rehab facility, and I was told there was no problem. You'd think any facility like this would be well-equipped with computer services." I am on a rant. Am I in computer withdrawal? Unwired taking on a new meaning? Then, I realize that these facilities are mostly inhabited by people ten years or more my senior, people who are not dependent on the internet the way I am. But from my generation forward that just won't be true. Hotels have caught onto their customers need for WiFi connections in their rooms, and many chains charge for the connection making up for their lost telephone revenues as their customers use their own cell phones. So, probably when nursing homes are wired, they'll add a user's fee, too. Oh Laurel! Stop being so cynical.

'You're right," Brandon says. "Our WiFi should be better. I'll try another way of connecting you. Any other problems?"

"Hello, Mrs. Richardson," an East Indian voice. "I am Prem. I will be your physical therapist today." He looks somber and sad.

"Where's Colleen?" I ask. I feel apprehensive.

"She's in school, today." Prem wheels me out of the room, without saying another word.

"Come and visit me later," Renee says in her throaty way. She's in the corridor. "I want to tell you something."

"Be glad to," I say.

We pass Trevor, who appears to be asleep in his wheelchair and enter a crowded Therapy Room. Prem sets me up on the NuStep.

"So, do you have plans for the week-end?" I ask Prem, although it is only Tuesday. The question is a standard one staff ask each other. Maybe I'm stepping outside my boundaries, but maybe I can start a conversation.

"No," he says.

I wait. This is an interview technique I use in my research work.

"No?" I repeat, another interview technique. I wait. I am good at waiting.

As if a gate has been opened and the flood-water released, Prem tells me he might get a phone call from his wife. She and his two sons are back in India visiting her parents. They have been there for three months. Traveling back and forth is expensive, and it is good for his sons to spend time in their homeland.

"It's hard, isn't it, to be separated," I say, feeling a little foolish, overly personal and invasive, after saying it.

"It is the right and good thing," Prem says. "So it is not hard."

"You don't have occupational therapy, today," Rhonda says. She's running in place. "Effie Lou's had a home problem. Again." Rhonda rolls her eyes. "So you can wheel yourself back to your room. Right?

"Hi, Renee," I say. I am proud that I maneuvered the corridor and wheeled myself into her room.

"Did you know that I have top security clearance in the Energy Department?" she asks me.

"Yes, Ernest told me."

"What all did he say—about me?"

Is she interrogating me?

"That's all. And that he was sorry this had happened to you."

"When this happened to me," she says, looking at her absent legs, "they retired me. Just like that. That's not right, is it? I've worked for twenty-five years for the Feds. I know a lot. Senators have wanted me to go to Washington—with my top clearance and what I know but I had family here, so I didn't go. Now, look at me."

Jingle-jangle.

"Here's your lunch—Lily and Bashi," Vena says in her lilting West African accent. She is softly humming *Jesus Loves You*.

"You're just great," I tell Vena.

"You can tell my children that."

"I've been through children problems," I say. "How old are they?"

"Let's see. One is eleven, one is twelve, and one is thirteen. All girls."

"I have three daughters, too," Ernest says.

Vena shrugs.

"Guess I'll take Lily and Bashi outside," Ernest says.

Vena picks up the tray and appraises me. "It's hard to keep exact track of their ages," she says. "We seldom talk."

"Do they like school?" I ask.

"How would *I* know, Miz Laurel." Vena's voice gets edgy. "They're in Sierra Leone with my mother."

"Oh. That must be hard." I can't imagine how painful this would be.

"No. It is better this way."

"Your work-schedule is erratic, I know." I wonder how parents in the service end of the health profession manage their careers and their families.

Vena looks at me with exasperation, a "what-the-hell-do-you-know" look.

I wait.

"I don't want them here because I don't want them in *your* middle-schools—exposed to *your . . . .*" She stops herself and abruptly leaves.

"Renee stopped me on the way back," Ernest says.

"Did she want Lily again?"

"Yes and me, too. She said she didn't know how you let me out of your sight. She said that I was a 'devil.' "

"Well, she's not right about that, is she?"

Ernest makes his fingers into horns and wags his tail.

"Whistle-A-Happy-Tune." That's my cell phone. My brother, Barrie, is the only one who routinely calls me on it.

"Hi, Honey," he says. "How are you feeling?"

"I'm good, and you?"

"We're just back from Des Moines," he says. "We've been to see Paul."

Paul will be 84 next week. He and my sister, Jessica, had been married for nearly sixty years, when Jessica died just short of her eightieth birthday. When they were high school sweethearts, I was the seven-year old pest spying on them, the "smarty-pants" solving algebra problems before they could, the little fraud who would accept Paul's nickel to "get lost," and then hide under Father's red leather chair where I could see them, but they couldn't see me.

Paul was a Marine on Pork Chop Hill in Korea, the only member of his platoon to survive. He returned frostbitten, sterile, and with uncontrollable rages and an insatiable need to control. He married Jessica, finished college, taught middle-school social science. I was the nasty "know-it-all" who earned a PhD in Sociology, while Paul dropped out of graduate school. I'm not sure if the worst thing I did in his eyes was to give birth to sons or to witness him abusing my sister.

Thirty years ago, Paul began sleeping on the living room couch; my sister began sleeping on the living room floor by the couch, like a dog. Twenty years ago, Paul was diagnosed with congestive heart failure, ten years ago with renal failure. His illnesses controlled my sister's life—and her dying. She monitored his salt and water intake, his medications, his doctors' appointments and twice weekly IV infusions. Both of them were in denial about how ill my sister was, about how much pain she was in from lung, colon, and breast cancers—all diagnosed in late stages. Only after my sister spent six hours unable to get herself off the floor and out of her soiled mess, did Paul accept her need for hospice.

I came at once. But Paul insisted that Jessica's "first rule" was "to get well," and her second rule was "to eat." She was in horrible agony for five days. He restricted her pain-medications, denying her the energy to attend to the spiritual tasks of dying—finding meaning in her life and death. She was never out of pain, never allowed to tidy up her life, forgive herself and others. And Paul? Paul turned his anger and loss toward me—swearing at me, throwing things at me, and denying me the right of partaking in my sister's final minutes of life or to see her body after her spirit left. As a final blow, he insisted that her body be given to science and that there be no memorial service.

Four years have passed since my sister's death, and I am still angry. I have talked about my pain and anger with Ernest, friends, and my grief counselor; I have written about it, made an art book, and two quilts; I have become a hospice volunteer working with bereaved children; and I have stopped telephoning or making plans to visit Paul. None of these pro-active choices have worked. It is as if I have hit a wall. I don't know what to do to eliminate the negativity I feel about Paul.

"Paul fell in the bathroom, couldn't get up and got dehydrated," Barrie tells me on the phone. "They took him to the hospital and put him on dialysis. At the hospital, he was swearing and throwing things at the nurses. They had to restrain him. He's in critical-care now with full-time nurses but he throws his food at them." Barrie pauses. "The doctor has had the 'preparation for dying' conversation with Paul, and

Paul has signed the 'Do Not Resuscitate' document. The doctor told Paul he has six months to live, but behind his back he held up three fingers and made sure I understood that Paul only had three months." Barrie pauses again. "Paul will have to be on dialysis three times a week... his life depends on it."

"He told me, he'd never go on dialysis," I say.

"Well, he's on it."

How ironic, I think, that Paul and I are both in facilities. I fall asleep, reading one of my purloined dog books. A dog with a collar feels proud, the dog narrator says, because he is an owned dog. I wonder if my sister...

I wake up thinking about Paul. When my sister was dying in hospice, an exhausted Paul would yell in his sleep. "I can't do this... Yes, I can... I can't... " I didn't know if he was yelling about Jessica's dying or his living through Pork Chop Hill, or both. No matter the horror, Paul holds onto his life. He doesn't want to die. His life-urge is intense. My sense of myself is that I would not fight if my life were challenged; that I would just give in. I don't think I would go through rounds of chemo or massive invasive surgery. I don't think I could tolerate what Paul tolerates—excruciating back pain, infusions, dialysis, a regimen of medicines, a dead spouse, a failing heart.

My anger dissipates.

I find myself admiring Paul—his will, his clarity. *Quality of life* is not the issue for Paul. Just being alive is.

What's this? What's happened?

Sinister, awful, treacherous Paul has become heroic in my eyes. The good vs. bad dichotomy has dissolved.

L'Chaim—to life. He chooses life. Will I?

January 11

According to brain researchers, two things are true when people have new and surprising insights. These things were true for Newton, Archimedes, Einstein—and now me, and everyone else who has ever lived and solved an intractable problem. First, you feel as if you have "hit a wall," around an issue or problem. You have exhausted your resources for solving it. You are so done. So, you turn your attention to something else like sitting under an apple tree, taking a bath, going to sleep. And, then the insight comes. But more comes. What comes is the certitude that your insight is correct. You don't have to prove it. You just *know* it. You know you are right. I *know* the insight I had yesterday about Paul being a "hero" is right. I can admire him, and move on.

"Got a surprise for you today," Colleen the p.t. says, sashaying into my room later than usual.

"Is that a scooter?" I ask. "For me?"

"It's called a turning leg caddy, actually," Colleen says. "But you ride it kind of like a scooter. Our manager has lent it to you... You put your bad leg up on the seat, bent at the knee, and push as jolly well you can with the good leg. It has hand-brakes like a bike. It'll be a lot easier for you to maneuver."

When I was nine, Paul taught me how to ride my new Schwinn bicycle. I balanced well and went riding across our back yard, an ersatz basketball court. But Paul neglected to teach me how to brake. I hit the garage wall, mangled the front wheel, and lost my pride.

Now, Colleen helps me onto the scooter, shows me to how to steer and brake. Off I go. I can get out the door by myself and whiz down the hall. "Hi, Trevor," I say, as I whoosh past him. I feel like a little girl, free and beautiful, zipping down this corridor that could be any corridor in the whole world. Zoom!

"Wait for me!" Colleen shouts, her redhead-Irish temper erupting.

"Hello, everyone," I say to the staff and patients in the Therapy Room. Look at me, look at me!

"Humph," says Violet. The long-term resident snaps her pop-beads at me.

Rhonda is doing squats by her desk. An angry looking dark-haired woman fusses with her foot brace. She can't get the Velcro to hold. "Someone help," she demands in a German accent.

"You have to learn to do it by yourself, Ilsa," Rhonda says without looking at her.

"Well, jes lookie you," says Effie Lou to me. Her eyes are puffy.

Jingle-jangle.

"Yap. Yap."

"Yap-Yap-Yap."

"Ernest," I shout, riding my scooter into the hallway. "I'm here. Therapy was later this morning. Bring Lily and Bashi in here."

"Puppies!" Heavy-set Effie Lou gets down on all fours to play with the dogs. She rubs their backs and scratches behind their ears. "Pap-pee-yons?"

"Yes," I say. "Bashi and Lily. Bashi means a little bundle of joy in Japanese, and Lily means Love. So, you are surrounded now by joy and love."

"I kin use all the lovin' I kin git," Effie Lou says. She gets up, sits on her stool and picks up Lily, who nestles into Effie Lou's ample lap. Bashi does a "stay" on the floor. "Ah have a two-year old Pug," she tells Lily and me. "Named him Squirt."

"Is he house-broken?" I ask. Pugs are known to resist training.

"Oh, I use pee-pads."

"Bashi came with those," I say. His breeder said he might spray in his new house to claim his territory, but he didn't.

"My husban' Tony's got a Pit bull, but he haz to keep it at his ma's house. Thaz where Tony lived before we got married. At his ma's with the Pit bull. I don't wan'any Pit bull in my house. Squirt don't like him. I don't trust him. I wanna 'nother dawg, though."

"Two dogs definitely better than one," I say. "They keep each other company."

"I wanna teeny dawg, like one of y'alls. I'm lookin' at a Yorkie-poo I saw online."

"What does Tony think about that?"

"Tony wants a Boxer. I tol' him, 'No Way! Ah'm the one's gonna clean up afta it. And buy its food. No way!"

I scoot back to my room with Lily, Bashi, and Ernest trailing behind. Brooke must have been here because my sheets have been changed, my commode emptied, my room neat and tidy, a glass of cranberry juice on my bedside table.

"Did Renee co-opt you?" I ask Ernest, when he and the dogs arrive some ten minutes later.

"Yep," he says.

"Yap," says Lily.

"She looked longingly at me, and asked if I had any friends who would be interested in a woman without legs. She took Lily on her lap and said, 'All my other parts are working.'"

"Poor Renee," I say.

"Yap," says Bashi.

For many years I went to First Unitarian-Universalist Church. I taught pre-school, met Ernest at one of the retreats, and sang for a dozen years in the choir. Many of my friends belong to the Church and some of my favorite women's groups—Memoir Writing, Artist's Way, Cakes for the Queen of Heaven, Women's Liberation—have their origins in the Church. But, about ten years ago, I began to pull away from the Church-as-Church: My spiritual needs were not being met as a kind of absolutism had settled into a secular litany. The referencing name changed from "Liberal Religious" to "Religious Liberals." Deleted from our "Mission Statement" were any words that might offend the humanist or atheist contingents—now the majority of the membership. Gone were "soul," "spirit," and "divine." I dropped out of choir and stopped going to church services and events. So, I was surprised when the minister Mark came to see me a few days ago, but even more surprised by how much I was looking forward to talking with him.

Ernest and the dogs had already left when Mark arrives. He looks exhausted, pale and puffy, and soft and sad. He comes from an Italian American family, was raised Catholic, but left that church because of doctrinal differences. His mother died a month ago. He lives alone in a loft-style condo near downtown. He has space for his art studio.

"I am so glad you're here," I say. "I'm so sorry about your loss of your mother."

"We learn so much we may not want to learn when a loved one dies," Mark says.

I tell him about my sister's painful death and about Paul's being out-of-control.

"How differently each person handles death," Mark says.

I tell him how Paul refused to let go of my sister—let her die—and how he began maligning my father—denigrating him while my sister twisted in agony—telling stories making my father a liar, a braggart, and totally useless around tools. That was particularly infuriating to me because my father prided himself—not on his successful legal career, service in the Cavalry or helping the "downtrodden"—but on his "puttering" around the house, fixing windows, framing pictures, making me doll furniture. Some of my happiest memories are hearing my father singing in his Irish tenor, "*It's so nice to have a man around the house.*"

"When we hear new stories—true or untrue—we are thrust into emotional chaos," Mark says. "Sometimes those stories bring us closer to our loved ones. That's what happened for me with my mother before she died. The stories she told me. I understood her better."

"Maybe, I'm understanding the living better," I say. "Maybe, I'm understanding Paul better—his anger and defensiveness."

I find myself relating a story. "A man shot a corrupt policeman to death. Immediately after the shooting, the murderer called my father asking him to be his defense lawyer. Father told the man to go to the Addison Avenue police station where he would meet him and they would schmooze with the coppers giving the murderer an air-tight alibi. The corrupt policeman was Paul's uncle—his father's twin-brother. Father told Paul this story the first afternoon they met.... And, Father told this story often with great gusto, his Irish eyes smiling."

"Quite a story," Mark says.

"Talking to you now, my mind is reeling. I've had a revelation." *I'm not sure I've ever used that word before. Revelation.*

Mark adjusts his glasses and sits back further in the chair.

"My father opposed my sister's marriage to Paul, not only because he was Catholic but because, I think, he believed Paul lacked drive, ambition, and came from an inauspicious family background. Paul proved him at least partially right by dropping out of graduate school and spending his life teaching middle schoolers. When the marriage progressed without a child, Father asked them to adopt a baby boy that Father knew came from a 'good family.' Paul refused."

Mark leans forward.

"Paul must never have lived up to my father in my sister's eyes," I say. "No wonder Paul's rancor and unremitting verbal assaults on my father."

"So much to take in at once, Laurel."

"Paul must have demeaned my father for years," I realize. "Not just when my sister was dying. It's just that I hadn't heard him doing it."

"Sounds like he never won that war," Mark says.

"Since my sister's death, I have seen Paul as villainous," I say. "But yesterday, I had an *aha* moment. In my eyes he became heroic because he has chosen life, over and over again, despite unremitting odds and suffering. I don't know if I would."

"When you open your heart and mind, Laurel," Mark says, "all manner of unexpected thoughts become possible, like seeing Paul through your sister's disappointed eyes."

"How sad that must have been for both of them," I say.

"And how defensive Paul would have to get."

I can't help but wonder about my father's expectations for me...

I know he thought I was too pugilistic, boisterous, and energetic. When I was three and getting into fist-fights with boys, Father made a rule: I was to measure myself next to the opponent. Only if I were shorter, could I fight. "Not fair!" I would scream. "If you expect life to be fair, you'll never be happy," Father would retort, followed by, "A soft voice is desirable in a woman." He enrolled me in etiquette, theater and modeling lessons. To "finish" me he added fencing, swimming, and English-saddle horseback-riding. These were all the lessons he thought appropriate for the woman he expected me to grow up and become: a docile wife of a professional man, a mother of perfect children, and, before the arrival of a child, a fourth-grade teacher.

Sorry, Dad, I didn't meet your expectations, either . . .

"So, where are you now, Laurel?" Mark's voice beckons me.

"Oh. I'm going to write Paul a letter telling him how much I appreciate him," I say.

"That sounds like the right thing to do, Laurel."

I start to giggle. I feel so much lighter. A fun thought enters my mind.

"You know Tina, right?" I ask Mark.

"Yes."

"Well, she and I are talking about starting a God Group at Church. We imagine the protests against us from the Humanist Group and the Atheist and Agnostic Group—Oh, the riling up of the children. Being on the 6 o'clock news. *Church Defies God Group.*"

"I'd join the God Group," Mark says. "**G**ood **O**rderly **D**irection."

I nod. I've heard that acronym before, but I have no idea what it means—or is supposed to mean. That everything that happens is good and orderly? Or only those things that are "good and orderly" are God-directed? Good and orderly for whom? In what direction? And who judges?

To me "Good Orderly Direction" sounds just like *functionalism*—the sociological perspective that sees society as a system in which all its parts work together like *organs* in a *body* presumably to ensure health and stability. The "GOD acronym" applies functionalism to the spiritual realm. *Hello!* Functionalism as a perspective is limited, naïve, and elitist: It favors the status quo. The ways things are, are the way things are supposed to be—so, those who have power and money and control the society's institutions, norms and media are doing the *right* things for the good of the whole society. Some of them have to get advanced educations (like doctors and dentists) and take big risks (like politicians and entrepreneurs) so they receive greater rewards (more money, prestige, status) on earth than others whose *functions* are less…*functional?* Taken into the spiritual realm, the "chosen" not only get everything on earth, tautologically proving that they are the chosen, they will hit the big Jackpot of Heaven. But, if we look at it all from the God-side, what we have is a hipper way of restating the Neo-Platonist argument that all things have been decreed by God in a *hierarchical Chain-of-Being and that there are no mistakes.*

"So, Mark," I say. "In Alexander Pope's words, 'Whatever is, is right.' But how about an existential twist. *Whatever is, is. Right?"*

We laugh. I feel I have found a friend in Mark. We hug our good-byes, but I find myself searching my brain for God-Thoughts. I envy my friends who are *certain.* Some are certain that the only God that exists is the one we make-up and that when we die we become bacteria and stardust, returning to nothingness like the nothingness prior to the womb. Other friends are certain that there is "something"—not a "someone"—that creates small miracles every day and that death will bring on more miracles. Christian-identified friends *know* that there is a God who will grant them everlasting life with other like-minded Christians. New Age devotees and Hasidic Jews *know* their souls have been reincarnated, and will continue to be so until they learn the lessons they need to reunite with the Divine Source. All I *know* for sure is that I *feel* better when I imagine a *benign force* around me, protecting me, and that when I give up trying to control the world, that which I need appears.

"Hi, Friend." Tina's signature greeting. Tina is a new and young friend from my Artist's Way Group and my co-conspirator for a God Group. She and I frequently imagine groups we could create—Kiddie-Lit for Adults, Spirituality for Women, Simply Living for All. Her hair is pulled back in a ponytail. She is fresh-faced, smiling. Tina is a licensed social worker, massage therapist, reflexologist, gardener, labyrinth-maker and part-time Title 20 pre-school manager. She is the eighth born of twelve children. She's been divorced for two years. I have told her how I "got" Ernest by writing a list of what I wanted in a man, bury-ing it away and forgetting about it, being happy with myself by myself. Years after Ernest and I were married, I found the list tucked into an old daybook. Ernest had all the traits I had listed. I wish Tina could be my daughter-in-law, but I don't have a free son so I am encouraging her to Write-a-List.

"Brought you some gluten free soup and biscuits," Tina says, set-ting the food on the table. On both sides of my gene-pool, I am gluten intolerant.

"Something I can eat that will agree with me, nourish me," I say. "Thanks." I take a spoonful of the soup and feel the elixir of the God-desses rejuvenating me. "Mmm . . . mmm, good."

"Organic kale, onions, broccoli, brewer's yeast and purified water," she says.

I take a bite of biscuit and savor the crumbly texture.

"And rice flour biscuits with rice milk."

"Perfect!"

"Are you up for a mini-massage?" Tina asks.

"Oh, my, yes. This is a good time to dispel old toxins."

After Tina leaves, I sit in my bed looking out my window at the night sky, and I imagine the universe as a place of vast silence. Fifty years ago, I was in a totally sound-proof chamber at the Navy Postgrad-uate Institute in Monterey. The Monarch butterflies had returned to their pine grove, a wintering sanctuary for them, and the sound of their wings could cause tsunamis in Indonesia and Japan, but I could not have heard them anymore than I could hear the pin drop on the chamber floor or the ball bouncing on the wall above my head. Absolute silence is eerie and disorienting, unlike the sleuth silence we think we are in when we turn off our electronic gadgets, close the windows and look at the stars. If there is no sound out there in the universe, I wonder, do the stars get disoriented? And is the stardust from which I am made more disoriented than that of the Monarch butterflies? My mind turns to the afternoon at Blendon Woods when Ernest and I washed, sexed, and labeled Monarchs before releasing them for their three-thousand mile journey to a special place that they knew about without having ever been there. We were awestruck silent.

CHAPTER 5

Lo And Behold

January 12

"Good morning, Ernest," I say into the phone. "Will you do me a favor?"

"Of course, Darling," he says.

"Please bring the stationary that Linda R. gave me—it's in a blue box on the second shelf of the large book case in my study—and bring the Georgia O'Keefe card box—it's on the top shelf of the same book-case—and a calligraphy pen from my desk-drawer." I am glad that I know just where some things are.

"I'll bring your mail, too," Ernest says. "And a surprise."

I like surprises. Ernest doesn't.

"Good morning, Laurel." Brandon's voice. "How's everything go-ing?"

"Well, the internet is not reliable and I've been thinking about health care and what needs to happen. You're the business manager, right?"

"Assistant," Brandon says. I can't tell if that is false pride or baleful-ness in his posture. "I have my degree in management of rehabilitation and long-term facilities, with a minor in business."

I start lecturing. "The way to cure our health-care problems, im-migration problems, and economic problems is to increase the number of nurse's aides—accept immigrants who want to work as aides, train them, increase their salaries and benefits and give them opportunities to move further up in health care—or—drum roll, please!—to enter college in related fields!"

Brandon listens, and then says, "We do have a step-system here. State certified and skilled assistants do receive more money, but we could have more steps, more motivators."

As Brandon talks, I ponder my gall. I have been in this facility for a week.

"The rule book for these facilities is inches thick," Brandon says. "They are extremely regulated. Would you like to read one?" Brandon's tone is not rancorous, defensive, or snotty. I think he likes talking with me.

"No, thanks," I say.

"I'll try to get your internet working," Brandon says. "Thanks for your ideas. I'll look in on you later."

Jingle-jangle.

"Hey, you good dogs . . . up on the bed!" I command. "I have a surprise for you." I take what looks like a Ban deodorant container from my bedside dresser, unscrew the cap and reveal a tidy rollerball that dispenses moist peanut butter. I offer the rollerball to Lily, first, as she is the dominant dog, and then to Bashi. Both dogs lick the ball and are beside themselves with excitement over the treat. "It's all natural goodness," I say. "Just like you two."

"Here's your mail," Ernest says, handing me a stack of envelopes. "And your stationary boxes and, your surprise!" Ernest holds up a new painting—*Deer Creek Pass, Sedona.*

He has used the pigments I brought back from Roussillon to create a vibrant painting of one of our favorite hikes in Sedona, a hike on which we never see anyone else, a hike where I can lead the way pretending that I am alone and that I am the first person to scout the trail. The hike starts at the foot of an extinct volcano, passes a wateringhole, and climbs through scrub forest ending at a cliff overlooking Oak Creek Village. Seeing the painting gives me hope that I will be able to take that hike again—and, if not, I will still have it in my sights.

He's brought picture hangers and a hammer.

"It might be against the rules to put a nail in the wall," I say.

"To hell with it," Ernest says, hanging the painting where I can see it from my bed. "Better to ask for forgiveness than to ask for permission."

I think about how both Ernest and I have created art spaces in our heads, hearts and home since our retirements from academia. His "studio" is in the basement, atop his workbench; mine claims the rarely used guest room. I am still exploring different media, while Ernest, after a brief stint with creating "Wall-Charms" and penning designs on pottery has settled into painting pictures. In the six years he has been painting, he has won Best of Shows, First-Place ribbons, and Honorable Mentions too numerable to enumerate. He has also served as President of our Worthington Area Art League. *You rock, Ernest!*

My first art memory is from kindergarten when my teacher lambasted my tempera painting of my house because it was brown—a dull color, I guess—while I was delighted with myself for having represented the house's color perfectly. Then, there were the grade school years where our "research" was judged by how pretty we made our folders. I got all "A s." Then, came my freshman year in high school. Now, a poem insists upon forming:

Whatever happened to my Mondrian knock-off
That Miss Nolan sent to the art contest
For high schoolers?

Did the judge put all the entries in a cardboard box
Where they've been blending colors
For fifty years?

Or were they were put in manila folders with soft
Green labels, just in case
One of us
Became famous?

My Mondrian knock-off earned me a scholarship to the Art Institute of Chicago's Saturday morning workshops for high schoolers. I attended. But only one time. When I saw how talented the others were—they could see! they could draw!—I withdrew.

"Can I come in?" Renee wheels herself into my room.

"Sure," I say. "Brandon was here."

"Who's Brandon?" she asks.

"Assistant business manager. He visits me a lot."

"He never comes to see me," Renee's whining. "No one from this place cares about me. I am going to get out of here, and the sooner the better."

"I'll talk to Brandon about you," I say. "But now, come and see Ernest's new painting."

Renee wheels herself close to the picture. She stares at it, backs away. "I don't get it," she says. "I don't get abstractions."

"Those are rocks," Ernest says pointing to the multi-hued red cliffs. "And that's a pond....and those are reflections of the rocks in the pond...and those are trees...and that's the sky."

"I can't see it," Renee says, squinting. "I don't get it... But, I am an artist."

"Acrylics?" I ask.

"Oil," she says.

"I don't like waiting for the oil to dry," Ernest says.

"Come to my room and see one of my paintings...And bring Lily."

On Renee's side chair is a large and well-executed oil painting of a tiger cub. The cub looks full of life and ready to play. Its eyes are luminescent. Its paws are smooth. "You're really talented," Ernest says.

"I've not had *art* lessons, you know," Renee says.

Someday I will hike again in Sedona, but I doubt that Renee will ever be back in her studio. Her wild-tiger days are probably over, too

"It's a wonderful painting," I say.

"I could paint Lily, if you let her come to my house." Renee cocks her head and smiles. "The whole second floor of my house is my studio."

"I had a burgundy-colored virgin wool coat with a tiger-fur lined hood and cuffs when I was twelve," I say, ignoring Renee's request for Lily. "I was at Marshall Field's with my mother and I tried it on and it fit me perfectly. I promised my mother I would wear it for years—that I wouldn't grow—which of course I did."

What I don't say is that because I was the youngest in our extended family, I was the recipient of everyone's hand-me-down clothes. Even my brother's. There I am—maybe 18 months old—standing next to my "big brother" on our cement front steps wearing too-long dark pants and an oversized pullover sweater. The burgundy coat with the tiger fur was of my own choosing, never having been worn by others, a genuine "virgin" coat. I loved how the fur felt next to my face and hands...how the burgundy color gave my cheeks a glow...and how the fashionable princess styling gave me a little shape...

"What happened to the coat?" Renee chuckles. "I could paint Lily lying on it."

"I think my mother gave it to a 'deserving little girl.'"

"Do you want me to hang the tiger cub painting up for you?" Ernest asks.

"Would you? I asked my daughter to but good luck getting her to do it. You know, she's awfully busy."

"I'll get the extra hanger I brought," Ernest says.

Does Renee know that the tiger is on the endangered species list? That only those living in protected parks have a chance to survive?

"I think we'll get the internet problem solved," Brandon says. He is back in my room. "We're getting an outside contractor to re-wire the router. It's not just your room. It's the whole facility that needs updating."

"Thanks," I say. "Everyone thanks you."

Brandon see-saws from foot-to-foot. He spies the painting on the wall, walks up to it and says, "Wonderful painting."

Either I've not broken a rule or Brandon has no desire to enforce it.

"Dear Paul," I write in my finest penmanship on my finest stationery. "I appreciate your valor and will…"

After I finish my letter, I decide to call my cousin Barbara to tell her the news that Paul has perhaps three months to live. I haven't seen her since my father's funeral forty years ago. She calls me about once a month to chat now that she is widowed.

"Hi Barbara," I say. "I'm in the rehabilitation facility…"

"Don't talk," she says. "And don't interrupt me."

"Okay," I say, surprised at her tone. Is she going to lambaste me for not calling her immediately about Paul?

"I read the story you wrote about camp and the lies you told," she spits out. "You have hurt me and I can't sleep. I can't believe you would say those things about my father…. You were such a sweet little girl… All I can figure is that you have something wrong in your head… that you have a brain tumor… or you're nuts… I can't sleep…" The lambasting goes on for twenty minutes about an article I wrote twenty-five years ago. The article was about being a child of a "mixed marriage"—Jewish mother and Protestant father—and took place in a Protestant family camp that my family and my gentile relatives went to every summer. Barbara is from the gentile side of my family. The internet had made the article available beyond my academic community.

"Are you still there?" Barbara asks.

"Yes," I say.

"Well?"

"You told me not to interrupt you, so I haven't."

"I can't believe you wrote this, Laurel. Are you sick in the head or what?"

"Barbara," I say. "I wrote the piece twenty-five years ago for a special audience. I told my truth. I changed every name and identifier of everyone. The last thing I would want to do is to hurt you. I am so sorry."

"Your mother was a saint. A goddess. You besmirched her. How could you?"

"I told the story," I said. "By the end of the story, she *is* a saint."

Barbara goes on, apparently not having heard what I said. "You treat your father like he is a prince. Well, he wasn't. He came on to the women at camp. He womanized."

"Yes, I talk about that in the article."

"He was a pervert."

"What?" *Tit-for-tat?* In the article I imply that Barbara's father was acting inappropriately with his youngest daughter.

"Your father was a child molester," she yells into the phone. "He took my little sister out in the boat and put his hands up her dress."

I am too flummoxed to ask "when" and too flabbergasted to say, "Everyone knows your sister was a little liar. When she lived with us—which she did for nearly a year, I don't know why—she lied about setting a fire in our attic, she lied about letting our dog out of the yard, and she lied about cheating on her homework. The neighbor kids sneered at her, 'Liar-Liar, your pants are on fire.'" Well, maybe they didn't. Maybe only I did.

The classic ethical dilemma that confronts qualitative researchers has confronted me: When you write the "truth" as you understood and experienced it, how do you shield the *Others* in the story from getting hurt?

"You lied over and over," Barbara says. "My father didn't drink Jack Daniel's. He drank Seagram's Seven."

Why is Barbara focusing on this minor point, rather than on the main ones about her father—that he slept in the same bed as Cousin Margaret at Camp, and that Margaret named her horrendously deformed baby after her father?

"Barb," I say, reverting to my childhood name for her and giving up on trying to explain the nature of ethnographic writing. "I am so sorry for your pain. The story is about how it was for me as a half-Jewish child to be in a gentile world where I was expected to fully participate in the Protestant service."

"We never treated your mother as different," she says, sounding furious. "We were totally ecumenical. It didn't matter if you were Congregational or Presbyterian or Baptist."

"Barb, I am so sorry to have hurt you but I have something I need to tell you. Paul is on dialysis and may have only three months to live."

Silence. Perhaps tears. Talk about how her husband died.

"You are my cousin, Laurel, and we may never talk again but I love you."

"I love you, too."

January 13

"Here's your rice cereal and rice milk," Brooke says. She looks like she's been hit by a tidal wave, rumpled and unkempt.

"Are you okay?" I ask. "I've missed you." Brooke has been my dependable sweetheart of a nurse's aide.

She straightens my cover and bites her lip, holding back a torrential rush of tears, I think. Then she tells me her mother had surgery for a brain tumor. Thankfully, it was benign, but the surgeon could not get all of the growth. She will have at least two more surgeries. The very best outcome will be that her mother will be blind.

I think about my Grandfather, who had come from Russia through South America with "my" samovar on his back. He lived with us the first three years of my life. He was a fine watch-maker for the Tsar, and a jeweler in America. When his eyes went bad, he became a Chicago taxicab driver. He spent the last years of his life in the Jewish Home for the Blind. He held his great-grandson—my son Ben—close to his heart, felt his face, hands and feet and called him, *kindela*, the pet-name he had called me. If my grandfather had lived now, he wouldn't have been blind. He would have had his cataracts removed, as mine were two years ago.

Why didn't I worry about that surgery? Perhaps because it is so common and perhaps because I didn't—and still don't—consider it *surgery*. I don't list it on medical forms anymore than I list tooth extractions and root canals. Furthermore, cataracts absent me from personal responsibility: I didn't cause them. The tendency is inherited. By the time I had my cataract surgery both my siblings and both my sons had had theirs. I drove my sons to the eye clinics, waited, and drove them home. That's it. Someone drives you to and from the eye clinic. That's it. You can see. I sound defensive...

I could see. My eyes had been astigmatic and weak since early childhood. I depended upon how people talked and moved to remember them. Never faces. It was not until eighth grade, when I was sitting at the teacher's table so I could see the black-board, that my mother had my eyes examined. Vanity and aesthetic preference for my familiar impressionistic world kept me from wearing glasses except when I *really* wanted to see *something*, like a movie, a painting, or the highway. Corrected, my eyesight at its best was 20/50. Uncorrected, I was technically blind. But choosing to not-see and not having that choice are oceans apart. To "pass" as something devalued—poor, Black, female, blind—is not the same as *being* devalued day after day. Am I afraid that I will be permanently devalued—an aging woman with an unsightly gait?

When I was perhaps four or five, my mother took my brother, my sister, and me to hear Helen Keller. We sat in the front row of an outdoor amphitheater on Lake Bluestone. I thought she looked funny and I laughed at how her voice sounded. Mother admonished me. "Stop laughing and pay attention to the great woman who has overcome her challenges." Afterwards, we came up on the stage and Helen Keller took my hand and said she could tell that I was a "special girl" and would be a "very good and important woman some day." I don't remember her saying that, but my brother says it is so.

Brooke's mother may end up blind, and here I am trying to tie together strands of my sighted life. I am ashamed of myself. . . I miss my grandfather . . . He was the only warm hand in my childhood castle . . . I miss my sister . . . After my mother died, when I was not yet thirty years old, my sister was my surrogate mother . . . Brooke's mother may soon be blind, and I, following my cataract surgery, can see better now than I ever have.

I take Brooke's hand and pat it, just as I patted my sister's hand before she died, and maybe the way Helen Keller patted mine. Am I trying to comfort Brooke or to comfort myself?

"Look at all your mail," Brooke says. The stack that Ernest brought yesterday is on the round table, still unopened. "Shall I bring it to you?"

"Thanks, Brooke," I say. "And I am so sorry about your mother. Can you come back later and stay awhile?"

She smiles her "yes."

Lots of cards and a package! The package is from Carolyn, just the person I want to talk to. Carolyn is a fellow qualitative researcher who writes extensively on the ethical issues of publishing research about friends and family. She is my closest friend in that research community. But, first I open her gift. How so like Carolyn!

I phone her.

"Hi, Laurel," Carolyn says with her distinctive Shenandoah accent. We share a love of that region, too. Ernest and I have hiked there, gotten lost in the woods there, and survived the roaming bears there. Both my ancestors and Ernest's ancestors had settled there; some are buried there. If they had stayed there, Carolyn and I might have been cousins instead of what we are: sisters in spirit.

"Thank you! I love those socks you sent with pictures of Papillons on them!"

"Thought you would…" Carolyn has two dogs, too, and she's been one of my go-to people with my dog questions. "…you're welcome…my pleasure."

We chat a bit about her research with Holocaust survivors and my ankle surgery, and then I ask if she remembers my article called "Vespers."

"I do," she says. "I teach it in my writing class. It's about your mixed-religion background and your problem adjusting to a Christian family camp."

"That's the one," I say, and go on to tell her about my gentile cousin lambasting me for what I wrote and how bereft I am over the rift.

"It's really hard, I know. Hard to weigh what's more important, almost impossible to succeed in disguising people, impossible to know who will see the work and how they'll interpret it."

"With the internet, I think we have to assume that whatever we write is public knowledge."

"You're right."

"I also feel confused and angry," I say. "My cousin said my father was a pervert—a child molester."

"That's one of the unspoken risks of writing about family … you might find out things you don't want to know."

"Or hear things that aren't true … and then you've got to deal with it."

Too tired to deal with it now …

"Laurel? Are you awake?" Brooke has come into the room.

"I'm glad you're here, Brooke," I say, opening my eyes.

I want to open my greeting cards. If I were to open them alone by myself somehow it would feel as if I were celebrating a birthday or a New Year alone. In the midst of all the plenty, I would feel lonely and sad. "Can you stay awhile?" She nods. Opening the cards with Brooke looking on, I feel that she is connected to the "me" at the Bellemont and to the "me" outside the Bellemont. I feel bonded to her in a celebration of life—hopefully, some of the messages in the cards will speak to her, too, ease her pain:

Granddaughter Shana's card is a woodcut of a woodpecker pecking on a birch tree—it says, "Perseverance, secret of all triumphs."

Bebe sends a card from my "Writers Who Read" group that has twelve mini-pictures of stick figures doing all manner of courageous things—climbing a mountain, straddling two chairs, jumping for joy—and saying "YES." The women in that group range in age from 72 to 88. They all live independently.

Thinking-of-you cards: two flower-cards from Jo, lilacs on one, a hand-painted red snapdragon on the other; a daisy garden from Deanne; a Williamsburg garden from Chris; Jeannie sends her water-color posies; Debbie sends me Snoopy; Amy, a dozen painted roses; Sophie, three grazing deer; a patriotic dog from Linda T; and from Joanne, who is recovering from a near-death medical emergency, "Chihuly over Venice."

Ernest and I were to go there last year, but my ankle prevented it…

Pat. L.'s card pictures a woman in a hospital bed with a great big comfy dog under her covers. "Hope you are back on your feet again soon." Because she connected us to Bashi and Lily's breeder, we consider Pat their Godmother.

A beautiful eight-point star quilt pattern from Carol, who wishes that "all my pieces be stitching together well."

Roger sends a card with a miserable angry-looking wet cat in a bubble-bath in a bathroom sink. Inside it says, "See, someone knows how you feel."

Get well cards—from Ben and Tami; Barrie and Janie; Chessie, my friend from toddler-hood; from Elaine, "May the sun warm you and the moon restore you and may the stars light your path to feeling better soon"; from Linda R., the Apache blessing of sun, moon, rain and breeze; a picture of a pitcher of tulips from Linda M. and Brenda; thirty-four signatures from the Discovery Group.

A turtle with a huge Ace-bandage across its shell from Nancy. "It's not the speed that matters. It's the getting there."

Three cards from Ellyn! A Chihuahua in bed with a thermometer in its mouth. "You'll be back on your paws in no time!" An Irish Setter driving a pick-up truck saying, "Thought you might need a lift!" A pudgy toddler boy with black sunglasses and leopard-skin patterned swim trunks stretched out fetchingly on a towel on a beach, reading a book. He looks like an Elvis love-child. "How're *you* doin'?" he asks. Julie, my outrageous Aussie friend, sends an outrageous picture of a woman in high heels sitting on a high stool. Her skirt is lifted showing her legs in rolled-down nylon hose. "It's you," she writes inside, "next year!"

My last PhD student, Carla, sends a purple card with a smartass little kid saying, "We've been through a lot together and most of it was your fault."

One-hundred and forty-nine signers on the "Circle of Support" card from First UU. I am surprised that I recognize nearly all the names, and can see in my mind's eye what the signers look like.

"Shall I put the cards up on your bulletin board?" Brooke asks. She pins them up and I see a menagerie, a bouquet, a collage—a visual display of that which cannot be seen—

No card from Cousin Barbara.

CHAPTER 6

You Have A Lot Of Friends

January 14

I wake up naturally—no knockings on my door, no moans of despair or snorts outside my door, no clatterings in the hallway. The sun is just waking up, too—and the glow on the snow gives a luster of midday to the courtyard below. I am atop my bed, still in my body, but with my spirits soaring—up on the roof top. This could be my Christmas morning.

More than two dozen greeting cards are pinned to my bulletin board—so many they have to overlap. How lovely to think of my friends "overlapping," and then to think of the many different circles of friendship I do have—university, art, writing, memoir, family, Discovery Group, church. Within those circles, there are smaller non-intersecting ones. Some of my friends are not in a particular circle, but in "my" circle drawn wide from across the Atlantic to across the Pacific, from Los Cabos to Alberta—and drawn long, from the seven-plus decades of my life.

I have written some about women's friendships, particularly about my best friend, Betty, who died from emphysema. If she were alive today, she would be hanging-out with me at the Bellemont. What I am feeling, though, is not the loss of my friend, but the pleasure I had knowing her. A cliché? Maybe.

A wondrous thing about friendship is that all societies across time and space have it, and in all societies the basic elements of friendship are the same: mutual aid, need-based helping, positive affect, gift-giving, and informality. Friendships are possible across cultures, genders, social classes and roles in places like the Bellemont—maybe especially in places like the Bellemont because of the proximity, ease of meeting-up and the freedom to let one's guard down. Almost like being back in college.

All that said, there are some times when friendships fracture and cannot be mended. One of those fractures has to do with *aging*—mine and others. It is harder to have active friendships with people who are in different life-stages. People who are raising children and building careers are in different spaces, have different interests and energies than those who have retired from childrearing and employment. After I retired, many of the women in my theory reading group took on administrative posts at the university. University politics dominated our reading group's discussion. My life veered from theirs.

Aging affects age-mates, too. I remember being mystified by Ernest's mother not seeing her best friend from grade-school because they lived thirty miles apart. Both women in their seventies, neither woman willing/able to drive the distance. Now, I understand it. I rarely see some women with whom I have been friends for decades. We've aged. Our energy is less. It takes longer to do everything. They've moved. They're ill. Their life-partners are ill. Priorities have changed. Grandchildren. Taking care of family, getting one's life in order, paradoxically, as one prepares to leave it, making meaning through self-reflection. It is not *as if* we are no longer friends. We still are, but we enact it differently—emails, occasional Skype, phone-calls, and a flurry of those when one of us is in an emotional chaos.

A magazine article I read when I was a teenager comes back into my mind. It has stayed with me all these years, because when I read it, I couldn't imagine feeling the way the writer did. The writer—a woman in her sixties—said she had moved from New York City to Staten Island and that she was grateful she had because she no longer wanted to have casual friendships or conversations. Living out of the city protected her from those time and energy drains. I understand that article, now.

"I have trouble phoning people nowadays just to say 'hello' and see how they're doing," I said on the phone to my friend Ellyn. She is nearly a decade my junior. She lives alone.

"I do, too" she said. "My days are busy. At night, I just want to be quiet, pet Surreal, eat my supper, read."

"In the daytime," I said, "I like to conserve my time and energy for writing. In the evening, I feel tired and I don't want to be taken into different people's lives. I don't want new things coming in, but I feel bad about myself, like I'm not being a good friend . . . like I'm a fallen angel."

"I feel the same way," Ellyn said.

"One of my college roommates whom I thought had died forty years ago was on my answering machine a few months ago." I said. "We had been friends . . . We saved each other's lives on one of our perilous canoe trips in northern Michigan. But I haven't called her back because I imagine we'd be on the phone for hours catching up, and I just can't find the time to do that. Ridiculous!" I paused and Ellyn waited for me to continue. "It is like how I feel about writing poetry, oddly enough. I can only intentionally write poetry when I feel I have unfettered time— not just hours, but days because I don't know where the poetry will take me emotionally. I guess I am afraid that if I phone my undead friend, it won't just be the hour or two on the phone, it might be taking me back into old college feelings that I don't want to have right now. I just want to write."

"Email her," Ellyn suggested.

"A good Saturday morning to you," Brooke says, coming in bearing my rice cereal breakfast, stolen fruit, and cranberry juice. She looks less rumpled today.

'How's your mom?" I ask. "I imagine she's very tired from the brain surgery?"

"She's resting." Brooke straightens my covers.

"Please give this greeting card to her." I had written a note of appreciation in it about Brooke's care-taking, and how proud I would be if she were my daughter. The last time I wrote to a mother I did not know was after the suicide of one of our graduate students. That mother called to thank me. This was a quarter century ago, and I still remember it. When my friend the spontaneous poet Mary Rumm was in hospice she gave me a similar gift—"Your son, Ben," she said—and then spoke out a rhyming sonnet about the teen-aged Ben's kindnesses to her, carrying her groceries, refusing a tip. This was a quarter century ago, too, and I still remember it.

"Perform random acts of kindness..." is a popular bumper sticker. And people do. It is a veritable social movement dedicated to the idea of doing kindnesses without any expectation of reciprocity. People drop coins at random near parked cars, give roses to passersby, offer free hugs. These are nice things to do and fit right in with our Tweet-culture. Welcome to Mackindness. But these nice acts, as nice as they are, cannot replace the *intentional* acts of kindness targeted to a *specific* person such as a neighbor, co-worker, club associate. These intentional kind acts weave together and mend the social fabric; it is these acts which make a community possible. These acts enrich the time spent in places like the Bellemont. How special it is when a staff member brings you cranberry juice out of "the kindness of their heart," as my mother would have said.

When I was a little girl, my mother read me a version of Aesop's fable about a mouse and a lion. A mouse awoke a lion from a sound slumber and so the lion threatened to swat him to death. The mouse pleaded for his little life saying that slaying a trifling mouse would demean the great and powerful lion. The lion agrees the mouse is measly and lets him go. A few days later, hunters snared the lion in a net of ropes. No matter how much he struggled, the lion could not free himself. The mouse heard the lion's roars and came to his aid by gnawing through the ropes. The intentional acts of kindness by the lion and the mouse toward each other saved both their lives.

Kindness toward others was the virtue my mother most valued. If I were planning a birthday party, for example, every girl in my class would have to be invited. It would be unkind to leave any girls out. If there was a child who was needy for friendship, I was to offer mine. It was the kind thing to do. If a child needed clothing, food, or money, then I should share mine. It was the kind thing to do. But there were limits. When I gave my rabbit-fur muff to a little girl I met on the El going to my grandma's house, I was chastised, not because I gave away my expensive muff, but because I gave it to someone I would never see again, a stranger, not a person in our lives. For strangers, what one did was raise money, knit scarves, fold hospital linens, or read to the blind.

When my mother was eight, she came with her mother to America from a stetl outside of Kiev. They escaped the pogroms; if they had stayed they would have been in a Nazi mass grave at Babi Yar. As Russian Jews in a new country, they depended upon other Russian Jews for intentional acts of kindness. Those acts built community with those they could depend upon. Reciprocity was a survival mechanism. Reciprocity saved lives.

What the Russian Jews did to survive in America—the construction of neighborhoods and alliances with people they could trust, people like themselves—is the same as every other dislocated or disenfranchised people have done, and continue to do. They establish networks of real and fictive kin to share the limited resources at their disposal. They live in the same neighborhood or housing complex. In Columbus, Somalian immigrants live either on the North or far Northeast side, depending on their tribal affiliation. Chin refugees from Myanmar have settled on the far west side. The African nurses and nurse's aides here at the Bellemont are mostly from Sierra Leone, and live on the near northeast side. We have areas of town called Italian Village and German Village, reflecting the ethnicities that settled them in the nineteenth century. Carol Stack's 1970 classic ethnography, *All our Kin,* laid out the complex rules around gift-giving in an African American housing complex. Single parenthood did not mean a dysfunctional family or need for a governmental welfare system. Reciprocity worked miracles. I taught that book in my gender, methodology, and theory classes.

Active adult communities, homogenous by age and childfree-ness, dot the landscapes of our southern states. I spent a month in one that offered organized activities from "A to Z." But, it wasn't for me. Rather than feeling a sense of peace, community and belonging, I felt the freneticness of my neighbors as they jumped from "A"—art, archery, archeology—to "Z"—zoology, zipper-repair, zoom lenses. I heard their golf and HDL scores. The deeper ties that bind were missing for me. I felt I had joined what Kurt Vonnegut called a granfalloon, a meaningless association of people. "If you wish to study a granfalloon, just remove the skin of a toy balloon," Vonnegut has written.

Now, I wonder about collecting the old and infirm in nursing homes. Can the proximity stimulate community? Or will the physical and mental limitations of the residents, combined with the desire for social disengagement, characteristic of those in pain or in the latter stages of their life, prevent it? People can be civil and neighborly, but is that enough to create strong bonds and deter loneliness?

Random acts of kindness are nice … but …

"Ready, Laurel?" my p.t Colleen has braced her back against my door. She is breathing with difficulty. "Let's have you ride your scooter … I'll help you get on it."

"Thanks … I can do it … "

"Hey. Look at all those greeting cards! You must have a lot of friends, Laurel."

"I do."

I scoot out my door into the hallway and notice that a throng of people are inside and outside of Renee's room. I am happy to see that Renee has a lot of friends, too. I scoot past Trevor. A well dressed woman—his wife? daughter?—is sitting beside him. She smiles at me. I scoot past visitors heading to the long-term wards and scoot my way into the Therapy Room, where Colleen puts weights on my "good" leg, and Effie Lou puts weights on both my good arms. "Hey, you all," I say. "Try as you may, you can't weigh me down."

I scoot out. Visitors are not in the corridor any longer, Trevor's alone again, and a man weighing perhaps three-hundred pounds is being transferred from a gurney into the room next to mine. A thin pretty woman—his wife I think—is bedside, looking relieved. I give her a little high-five wave. The throng around Renee's door has thinned.

Jingle-jangle.
Dog-nap time.

"How's the internet working? Brandon asks.

"Great," I say. Twelve friends have sent me good wishes. "Have you had a chance to check-in on Renee?"

"Not yet."

"Poor Renee!"

I think about her leglessness and Google "detached legs." I get 10,600,000 hits—"funny" street-art, "funny" YouTube videos, and insects, including a science video of a brown spider on a cutting board sitting beside her twitching detached leg, and for spiritual help, an Islamic dream interpretation of a the loss of both legs: loss of money and strength.

Poor Renee!

Tea-time! In comes my friend Carol toting a large bag from which she pulls out a hand-painted tole tray. She sets it on my bedside table and places two china cups and saucers, hand-embroidered linen napkins, a teapot in a tea cozy, gluten-free cookies, and a pot of miniature violets. Carol is a new friend from my Artist's Way group. Carol creates beautiful spaces wherever she goes. She sits on the bedside chair and pours us green tea. Her silver hair is cut short. She is wearing a sea green silk scarf around her neck, scrunched and tied, tails streaming to her jeans. She is a tiny woman.

"This is fantastic, Carol," I say, munching on a cookie.

We chat the way new friends chat—filling the other in on relationships and experiences that happened before the friendship took hold—or before one even knew there would be such a person in one's life with whom one could be friends. We chat the way new friends that trust each other chat—having no problematic history to ignore or mend. We chat the way new friends who have had similar heartbreaking experiences chat—glad to retell the story, glad to listen and to be heard. To be in my eighth decade and have a new friend in her seventh feels nearly miraculous.

"Do you need anything, Laurel?" Jamal asks. He has taken away my dinner tray, and is now walking around my room, a little like a caged animal or a basketball star.

"I'm good, thanks," I say.

Jamal keeps walking about my room.

"Have you had a chance to read the *Colonel Pettigrew* novel I lent you?"

"I—I have . . . ."

"So, what did you think?"

I wait.

"I thought the Colonel's friendship with Mrs. Ali was developed in a wry, unexpected, and completely satisfying way," Jamal says. "But the ending felt contrived."

"I agree," I say with enthusiasm. "The author wrote an unbelievable splashy ending—couldn't let a friendship just be a friendship."

A lovely Saturday evening surprise! My step-daughter, Deirdre, has come to visit with her two teen-aged daughters, Nadia and Vallia. I claim that I married Ernest for his daughter Deirdre, because there had always been a Deirdre in my father's family, and I like upholding traditions, but I didn't birth a daughter myself. If I had, I couldn't have named her "Deirdre" because Russian Jewish superstition carried forward from my mother's mother would have forbidden it. Jewish children are only named after deceased people, so that the deceased one can live on in another generation's memory. "What," she would have scolded, "you want my brother's daughter dead?"

"Hi, Grandma," Nadia says, leaning down to hug me.

"Hi Grandma," Vallia says, giving a brief hug. Both girls are dark-haired, green-eyed beauties. They dress in multi-colored layers, looking like dancers in a kaleidoscope. Nadia's signature style is mis-matched socks; Vallia's is barrettes and boots. They study dance and both are students at an Evangelical Christian school.

Their family had been missionaries in Petrozavodsk, Russia, a town some eight hours north of St. Petersburg by overnight train. Ernest and I visited twice. The first time, the family was living in a three-room basement flat in central Petrozavodsk. Filtering the water three times made it safe for washing diapers. Their entry was used as a public urinal. Russian doctors advised Deirdre to take her children outside for at least two hours a day, regardless of the weather, to clear their lungs.

On our second visit, the family had moved to a four-room, seventh-floor "suburban" apartment, "Stalin Arms." The elevator broke while we were in it, careening to the basement floor, where we waited for two hours for someone to let us out. Its backyard's dovecotes were filthy, unoccupied. A heavy iron gate and multiple steel key-locks guarded their apartment. Inside, cupboards rose from floor to ceiling. They held sterile medical essentials: routine shots, antibiotics, prescription pain killers, allergy medications, syringes, needles, ointments, bandages. Their kitchen looked like the separate kosher kitchen my grandmother kept seventy years ago in our south side Chicago "mansion": crazed porcelain sink perched on thin legs, zinc faucets, ceiling-high cupboards, small refrigerator with its cooling fan on top, old green stove, white porcelain-topped table.

A few months later, the family went on vacation. When they returned, nearly all their worldly possessions had been stolen—including the steel door. Pensioners who lived in their building had also been burglarized, and then murdered, as they had the misfortune to be at home.

Ernest and I were relieved when the family returned to Columbus. We celebrate their presence every Monday night with a "blended" family dinner. Ernest cooks for eight to twelve of us, depending. Nadia had the school assignment to write about her favorite day of the week. "Monday," she wrote, "because we go to Grampa and Grandma's house."

"How're you feeling?" Deirdre asks me. She takes off her coat and sits in Ernest's chair, the comfy one by the window. "Take off your coats, girls," she says. "Move the table and chairs closer to Grandma's bed."

I wonder if it is difficult for the girls to see me like this, leg wrapped up, body propped; I wonder if it is hard for them to visit in a nursing home, especially hard for Vallia, who buries her head and stops up her ears whenever dinner-table conversation veers to the gross or morbid, which happens often because the guys at the table tend to control the conversations about movies, news, politics.

"We would have been here earlier," Deirdre says, "but this is our first free night."

Saturday night—still a "free night" for these beautiful girls… but not for much longer. "So, you girls aren't dating?"

"Gross," says thirteen-year old Vallia.

"I would," says fifteen-year old Nadia, "if there were anyone I wanted to date and if my parents would let me."

"But we won't," says Deirdre. "There's plenty of time for that. Enjoy each year you're in."

I think about the year I am in…and where I am spending it…and about the aged and infirm that fill the wings here at the Bellemont…some, like me, to be rehabilitated and leave…others, not so…

In America, if we have the financial resources when we are older or infirm, we can hire home health-care assistants. We can move to one of those active-adult communities or a continuing care facility, stepping down from independence to assisted living to nursing care. We can live with an adult child, although that child is unlikely to have the time, energy, or skills to care for our medical needs. Many of them are of retirement age. They must feel resentment, wondering when they'll get their time to rest and relax in the sun. The sandwich generation, now an open-faced sandwich, the young-old taking care of the old-old. Or, we can come to a place like the Bellemont. If we are indigent, we can call upon Medicaid.

"What's wrong with being in a nursing home?" I had asked my Memoir Writing group last year. They said:

"It's the attitude in most of them. You get treated like a child with orange doohickeys put on your door for Halloween."

"You lose your freedom."

"You lose your privacy."

"Any pretense of individuality is erased."

"It's a downward spiral and you know it. You lose hope."

"The assault on one's senses, the smells, sounds, sights."

"I like taking care of other people, not being taken care of. My sense of worth would be damaged beyond repair."

"It's your final resting place before your final resting place, the cemetery."

"Is it better to be taken care of by your family?" I asked.

"No," they said. "Wouldn't want that burden put on them."

"Is suicide a better option?" I asked.

"Yes," said several, "if you can time it right."

I bring my mind back to my visitors. "So, what were nursing homes and rehab facilities like in Russia?" I ask Deirdre. She is a social worker with a case-load of senior citizens in and out of nursing homes. Part of her missionary work in Russia was with the elderly.

"Elder care in Russia is still seen as the responsibility of the family. There are almost no assisted living or rehab facilities. Putting your parent in a nursing home is considered shameful... Hospitals are deadly but nursing homes are even deadlier... Many are fire-traps... Help is insufficient, supplies are lacking—syringes and needles are reused—sanitary practices? *Nyet.*"

"I'd never put you in a Russian nursing home," Vallia says to her mother. Her voice is shaky.

"Thanks, sweetheart. But for aging women in Russia who have no children or whose children can't care for them, what choices are there?"

"I bet those women feel lonely," Nadia says. "I would."

"They do, honey. And frightened. Getting older is the biggest fear of Russian women… With age comes poverty, health problems, and loss of dignity."

Don't American women have these same fears?

"What about the men?" Vallia asks, wiping her tears.

"Oh, they die young… in their early sixties… mostly caused by high-risk behavior or alcoholism."

"Let's change the subject," Vallia suggests.

"How about dreams?" Nadia says. "I dreamed that Mom and Dad had another baby. A boy."

"Gross," says Vallia, sticking out her tongue.

"Well, that's not going to happen," Deirdre says.

"Good," says Vallia, looking half-relieved and half-nauseated by her thoughts. "We'd have to take care of it and everyone would look at us. Gross!"

"I can imagine having a baby brother," Nadia says. "But only after I am already grown-up and he's grown-up and in college. I can imagine helping him through college."

"That's nice," their mother says.

CLANG! CLANG! CLANG!

"What's that noise?" Vallia asks.

"It's the eleven o'clock closing bell," I say.

"Is it eleven? The time went fast," Nadia says.

"When you're having fun…" Deirdre and I say together.

This is the first time in over a year that I have spent extended time with Deirdre and her daughters without the guys around. We have talked like girlfriends do.

"Thanks for coming," I say, as they don their coats.

CHECK HALL 100 EXIT CHECK HALL 100 EXIT CHECK HALL 100 EXIT RRRRRRRRIIIIIINNNNNNGGGGGGG RRRRRRRRIIIIIINNNNNNGGGGGGG

"Can I come in?" Renee's whispery voice.

"Come on," I say.

"Look at all your cards," Renee says, wheeling herself in. "And all the people that come to visit you."

"You had a lot of friends visit today, too." I smile. "I was happy for you."

"They're family."

"That's nice."

Renee cocks her head at me. "I haven't seen most of 'em in years."

"Nice of them to come, then."

"Hmmf." She raises her eyebrows, pokes her head back down , and thumbs her knee. "They all have sob stories."

"Oh, I'm sorry."

"Don't be. They haven't come to see me… They've come 'cause they think my malpractice suit will get me lots of money… They want my money." Renee starts to cry.

"I'm so sorry, Renee."

"You're my only friend, Laurel. You're the only one I trust."

January 15

____

Sunday is "visitation" day—
Nancy
Josh and Akiva
Linda M. and Brenda
Ernest, Lily and Bashi

And phone-calls day—
Chessie
Linda T.
Maggie
Barrie
Shana
Cheryl
Elaine
Ellyn

Nan
Jean
Sarah
Pat
Patti
Patricia, pat … pat … pat …

And email day—
Carolyn
Julie
Nan
Lisa
Tami
Karen
Norman
Zzzzzzzzzzz . . . .
Zzzzzzzzzzzzzzzzzzzzzzzzzz

&

CHAPTER 7

Snake Pit

January 16

It is four o'clock in the morning, and I am awakened by the ear-blasting sound of my next door neighbor's television. I push my buzzer.

"Whazza mattah?" A voice I don't recognize. A scent of carda-mom.

"Can you get the television set turned down, please?"

"Prob'ly guy cain't hear so well."

"But I can!"

Unrecognized Voice leaves my room. The television keeps blaring. I push my buzzer again.

Twenty-minutes later, Vena asks in her soothing Sierra Leone accented voice, "Can I help you Miz Laurel?"

"The damn television set is too loud."

"He's new. He came in yesterday."

"Can you lower the sound?"

"Some people can't fall asleep without the television on."

"And some people—like me—can't sleep with it blasting on!" When I don't get enough sleep, I am short tempered.

"I'll see what I can do."

A few minutes later, there is silence once again.

"BLAH-BLAH-BLAH." A woman's piercing voice.

"BLAH-BLAH-BLAH-BLAH!-BLAH!" A man's penetrating voice.

It is 4:45 a.m. I can't stand it. How can anyone choose to listen to the banging anvil-heads on the television talk shows? What does this assault on one's ears and sensibilities do to you—day after day after day? How can it not contribute to illness of the body and soul? When we got our dogs, their breeder said we should leave the radio on all night for them so they wouldn't feel lonely. We let them listen to talk radio, until we listened to it, too. Why would we want our dogs' heads filled with human hostilities? We switched to the classical music station. Our dogs seem to sleep better. If only my neighbor had an FM radio . . . I push my call button.

"I turned it down," Vena says, anticipating my request. "But he must have turned it back up."

"What about closing his door?" I say. I put my pillow over my ears and imagine I'm listening to a Wagnerian chorus.

PUSH! It is five a.m.

"Yes, Miz Laurel?" Vena's come back in.

"Please try again. Maybe take his remote away. Maybe unplug his set. I can't sleep through that TV noise. "

"Here's your breakfast, Miz Laurel." Vena sets my tray on my table. "So, you got some sleep."

"Hmm?" I try opening my stuck-shut eyes.

"I fixed the problem," she says, looking ten feet taller. "I had his wife take away the remote."

"Good Morning, Laurel." Brandon, the Assistant Business Manager has come in. His hair is sheared close to his scalp. "How are you today?"

"Dammit! I'm mad!" I tell him of the television blaring away. "I'm exhausted."

"Many of our patients are hard-of-hearing," he says.

"Exactly," I say. "So, the facility should give everyone headsets or have enforced quiet hours or volume controls on the TV sets, like they do in motels." Obviously, in my precious few minutes of sleep, I had solved the problem. Solved it three-times over.

"We do have quiet hours between 11 p.m. and 7 a.m. I'll remind the nurses," Brandon says. "And we do have head-sets although we don't seem to use them. I'll see what I can do. And, I appreciate your feedback and suggestions."

"Oh... and I can't get my reading light to go on."

Ring. Ring. Ring.

"Hello?"

"Hi, Laurel. It's Colleen. Can you come to physical therapy in an hour?"

"Good plan," I say. "I'll take a nap now."

Ring. Ring. Ring.

"Hi Laurel. It's Colleen. Sorry, you can't nap—I'm ready right now for you—not later. Come in your wheelchair."

I transfer my tired body into my wheelchair and maneuver my way out my door. A tall haggard looking man of indeterminate age is standing by Renee's open door. He has the same coloring and head shape as Renee.

"Hi," I say. "Are you Renee's brother?"

The man recoils. "NO! I'm her father."

"Come and meet my mother," Renee calls to me. Her mother, a gray-haired tired-looking woman, is sitting by the large table. She is twisting the hem of her dark blue sweater with both hands, kneading it like bread.

"I'm her daughter, Miranda." A lithe brunette eyes me.

Had I told Renee that Lily was once named Miranda?

"And in the corner over there hiding over there is my granddaughter, Jody." Renee says. "Come on over here, honey. Meet my friend, Laurel."

Jody stays in her corner, lowers her head. Judging from her absent front teeth, she is five years old and is probably thinking 'if I can't see anyone, no one can see me.'

I make my way to the Therapy Room. Trevor's not in the hallway. I miss him. The room is full—Ilsa, the angry German woman with the foot brace; Violet, the angry long-term resident; several incapacitated men; several other women; and me. My new overweight next-door neighbor is stretched out on an extra-wide mat. Colleen sets me up with my weights and wig-wags her way to a back room. She returns with an African American woman in a maroon skirt-suit.

"Laurel, meet Johnetta," Colleen says. "Johnetta is the therapy supervisor." I am trying to remember whether it is polite to introduce the more important person to the lesser important person or vice-versa or if it even matters anymore and what constitutes importance nowadays and if Colleen would care about what Emily Post prescribes. But I am sure that Johnetta does.

"How do you do," I say to Johnetta. I know that is the polite response. I wouldn't want to annoy Johnetta.

"How do you do, Laurel." Johnetta skips the small-talk and goes directly to our business. "I have arranged my schedule so I can join you tomorrow."

"Thank-you!" I gush. Tomorrow, my surgeon, the wonderful Dr. Girard, will remove my wrapping and give me a walking cast. It's a big day of uncertainty for me. I appreciate that Johnetta will be there.

"Be sure to get an exact prescription from your doctor about your physical therapy," Johnetta intones. "Do not accept a general statement. It must tell us how to proceed."

"Johnetta," I venture. "Perhaps I could be given some Depends. I am a little worried about how long I might have to wait and whether there will be a handicap bathroom."

"You're going to a medical facility," Johnetta says. "They'll follow the American Disabilities Act. You won't need Depends." I feel dismissed.

Johnetta assesses my wheelchair. "It's large, but it will *probably* fit in the ambulette."

I wheel myself back down the corridor. Trevor is back, looking spiffy. He's had his hair washed and trimmed. The maintenance man, Gunther, is in my room fixing my reading light. He's muttering under his breath about the poor quality of the electric fixtures. "They put these darn things in when they remodeled this place thirty years ago—no, thirty-two years ago," he tells me. "They weren't any good then and they're worse now. It's time for another remodel."

"Will you do it?" I ask.

"I'm too busy rehabbing my church's fellowship hall." He grunts and picks up the broken fluorescent tube. "Well, that's done. Anytime you need anything, call."

"Hi, Renee," I say as I wheel myself past her doorway. "Your granddaughter is adorable."

"Do I look like a witch?" she asks, pointing to her hair.

"You couldn't look like a witch even if you were wearing a pointed black hat," I say. Renee's long brunette hair is falling softly around her face. Her skin looks smooth and soft.

"Then why won't Jody come to me? She acts scared of me."

I take the plunge. "Maybe she's a little unnerved by your legs being different."

"Do you think?"

Does Renee not know that her leg stumps disturb most everyone who sees them?

"Well what can I do about that?" Renee pouts. Her lips look like rose petals.

"Maybe when Jody comes to visit, you could put a blanket over your legs."

"You mean, hide 'em?"

"Just for now," I equivocate.

"Well—look at your hair." Renee changes the subject.

"Am I looking like a witch?" I ask.

Renee raises her eyebrows and nods her head.

"Well then I'd better go and get my hair washed right now."

I wave good-by and wheel myself toward the beauty shop. I am definitely stronger than last week and more confident. I wheel past the long-term Ward B. The Corridor Woman is grunting in her wheelchair. She *does* look like a witch. Uneven strands of oily gray and black hair spew from her head, as if she is in a Medusa cult. Doesn't anyone comb or wash her hair? The "Help me" man is on his back in his bed, moaning, and his roommate is slapping his own forehead. Killing demons? So many sick and old people here in the hallway. I come to the Activities Room, and say hello to the Director, who is at a table with two of the healthier long-term residents.

"Join us," a curly-haired woman says. "We're getting the Bingo game ready."

"Thanks," I say. "I'm going to the Beauty Shop."

"Well, stop by afterwards, then," a painfully thin woman says. "If you win, you get Bingo money to spend in the Bingo store." She is wearing a maroon-colored sweat-shirt from my alma mater, the University of Chicago, a bastion of progressive thinking. When the campus was built, its buildings were adorned with sculptures of *grotesqueries*. They are still there. A representation of one has been silk-screened onto Thin's sweatshirt. Monstrous likenesses of ethnic or racial minorities would not get out of the printer's press, but apparently disfigurement as adornment is okay on buildings and shirts.

"The store is open today!" Curly-haired gleefully spews out the news.

"What's in the store?" I ask.

"Good things," Thin says.

"Shampoo, combs, deodorant—toothpaste," says the Director—"stamps, things like that—things they need but can't afford to buy."

"Do you want your hair trimmed today?" Mildred asks.

"Just washed, pleased."

I decide to wheel back to my room the long-way, through Wings C and D to avoid another Bingo conversation. I plan to meet my Art League friend Randy's sister. I wheel into Wing C. Residents are not in the hallways, but their bed sheets are. The stench of urine and feces is sickening. The walls reek. This is the meme 'nursing home.' This is like being in Russia. How do the unskilled nurse's aides stand their work? I don't breathe until I have turned the corner into Wing D.

Wing D—Room 2060 has two beds. The woman nearest the door is catawampus on her mattress. She is wearing a red caftan and does not return my greeting as I wheel past her. Randy's sister is in the far bed, near the window. She is surrounded by boxes, books, and tschotskes. She could be on *Hoarders*. She looks like a female version of Randy, black and white hair. She is wearing several layers of white nightgowns. Her television is blaring away with a reality show. She is watching it and working on a crossword puzzle. I tell her I am a friend of her brother's and that I am in the rehab wing. She puts the TV on mute, but continues to keep an eye on the set, occasionally tapping her pencil on her in-progress crossword puzzle. She tells me she has seen my Papillons playing in the courtyard and that she likes looking at them. We have nothing more to say to each other. I feel like an intruder, a trespasser into this woman's private space. She wants to get on with her life—reality show, crossword puzzle. I want to leave. Neither of us has the gall to fake a friendship.

All the so-called space that surrounds people impacts how they feel and how they conduct themselves. Physically and mentally challenged people are even more intensely affected. How would I feel if I knew I were going to spend the rest of my life inside the Bellemont? Live in a long term ward? Share a bedroom with a stranger—or a series of strangers? A white curtain drawn between us the laughable nod to privacy? If I were "lucky" enough to be here the longest, I could have a window-side bed. I might see shrubbery, fences, walls, parking lots, jumble, yellow dumpsters, and sometimes a staff member, smoking. If I were new, my bed would be a few feet from a corridor that looks like all the other corridors here—same color, same railings, same glossy floor, same uninspired flower pictures hung too high for me to see from my wheelchair, my head crooked down? If I ventured away from my corridor by myself, would I get lost?

The Bellemont's space is not empty. It sends messages: fortress-like nurse's stations; boutique hotel-style main entrance; timeshare-resale look of the registration office with its brochures and green folders folded on its oversized desk; the Director's office, door always closed; the Therapy Room which does not welcome long-term residents; and the Activities Room, Dining Room, and Family Room shared by all residents, regardless of their differences in cognitive and physical functioning. Nowhere is there a nook or a cranny for privacy. The only warm and comfortable spaces seem to be for the adult-children, who will be choosing the new "forever-ever-after home" for their parent.

"I loved redesigning the interior of medical facilities," a friend told me. "I'd meet with the owners and administrators to see what they wanted. Then, we'd have an open meeting that the nurses and doctors were invited to. Doctors never came."

"What did the nurses want?'

"Beds! They were all about picking beds that were easier for them to adjust."

"What colors?"

"Mid-values."

"Did you invite the nurse's aides?" I asked.

"No. They were mostly temporary."

"What about the patients?"

"They'd be too diverse."

Temple Grandin, the high-functioning autistic animal scientist, knew from her own autism experiences how threatening and anxiety producing environments can be and how it feels to have those experiences denigrated and ignored. She describes herself as a "visual thinker," a person who can see details and replay what she has seen as if she is watching a movie re-run. This led her to design humane livestock-handling procedures that calm the cattle before their slaughter. Her work has received a Proggy award from PETA—People for the Ethical Treatment of Animals.

I think we need Temple Grandin re-designing our nursing homes. Wouldn't it be wonderful, if the redesign started with input from the lower strata—the long-term residents and their aides? But architects talk to The Client—the owners—not the users of the space.

I think about a recent conversation I had with my friend Carla—an architect and sociologist. She dashed my hopes for a remedied architectural practice and education.

"Doesn't the green movement tell the designers to stop thinking about medical environments as hotels, hospitality suites, or holding pens but as potentially healing environments?" I had asked.

"There's a green movement for certifying buildings," Carla said. "LEED—leadership in energy and environmental design. But it is all about consumption, what products to buy to check off the list so our buildings can get rated. It's not holistic or theoretical . . . or about healthy environments. It's like a politician wearing a flag pin. Green Patriotism!"

"Well, then, what about the New Age Movement? The Taoist idea of Feng Shui . . . The idea that the land is alive, full of *chi,* and that balancing the energy of any given space contributes to the health of the people living in it," I countered. "Surely all the young and hip architects know about that."

"No, they don't. It is not taught. It is not talked about. Really. Not at all. Never. Nowhere to be found in Western architectural schools of practices."

"Then what about the new hospital where I had my surgery?"

"Tell me about it."

"It was so Feng Shui. I felt so calm. Upon entering the lobby, I saw a path through gardens and beach rocks leading to a waterfall, and the soothing sound thereof. Next to a wall of windows, a brightly dressed volunteer stood beside a small lectern. Through an electronic communication device, she summoned a nurse's aide who arrived immediately, smiled, and ushered me into a private room, not an open-walled cubicle, for registration. Everywhere the colors were warm and soothing; no hospital grayed-green anywhere. The pre-op room is a room, not a bed separated from another bed by a curtain. After the surgery, I awakened in what felt like a regular bed in a nearly heart-shaped private room—my post-op hospital room, not another cubicle from which I would be transferred. Flowers were in a translucent vase, a gift from the hospital. Ernest was there, too, and several nurses. Staff talked to each other electronically, quietly. There were no clanging bells or paging messages or code blues. The P. A. system is used only when a baby is born. Then "Brahms' Lullaby" is played."

"Nice you had that experience," Carla said. "No doubt it was value-engineered for high-end patients with high-end insurance."

"Like me," I said, once again being reminded of my privileged life.

A Time For Every Purpose

January 17

"Are you sure the plans for my being picked-up are in place?" I ask Kiendra, the beautiful but unfriendly West African nurse. The hair-braid atop her head is gone. It is ten o'clock. Ernest is here without the dogs. I am sitting in my wheelchair with my purse and light blue fake-fur-trimmed parka on my lap.

"You worry so too much," Kiendra says looking at my wrapped-up leg. She smiles at Ernest, barely perceptibly pulling back her shoulders and asks him, "You drive you self in you own car?"

"That's the plan," he says.

Kiendra taps her foot, frowns, and turns toward the door. "Life-HealthCare will be here," she says. "I put the orders in myself."

"When?" I venture to ask.

"When I told them to come."

"When is that?"

"Soon."

"My appointment with Dr. Girard is at 11:00."

"You worry so too much." Kiendra flounces out the door, head held high.

"Hello, I'm Jim." He looks like an ex-wrestler, muscle gone to fat. "I'm from LifeHealthCare. This is Zoe." Tiny suntanned Zoe looks like Panacea, the Greek Goddess of Healing. It is 10:30.

"Hi, Jim. Hi, Zoe," Ernest and I say almost in unison to the odd couple.

Ernest helps me put on my jacket. Zoe puts on my gait strap, pulling it tight.

"We'll have to stop at the nurse's station to check you out," Jim says, pushing my wheelchair. "This is a big chair, but I think it'll fit in the ambulette."

Kiendra is doing paperwork. She shifts her eyes from Ernest to Jim to Ernest. She hands Jim a clipboard. "You must sign here," she says rhythmically tapping her index finger at the bottom of a page, "You must sign you name. You."

Jim pushes me down the corridor. Ernest follows behind.

"You must sign her out," the elderly Volunteer Greeter in her bright green vest says to Ernest, handing him a clipboard. "When will you be back?"

"We're going to the doctor's," Ernest says. "Who knows how long."

"Well, don't let it take more than three hours," she cautions. "That's the maximum Medicare allows a patient to be gone."

"Not if they're going to the doctor," Zoe corrects her. She sounds annoyed.

"I don't know about that," the Volunteer Greeter insists. "I'm just being helpful."

Jim wheels me to the door. Ernest holds it open so we can leave. I am anxious. I have not been outside for two weeks. I am unable to walk, and my strength is questionable. There is snow on the ground, and more falling. I feel vulnerable.

Jim wheels me under the forty-foot awning that ends at the curb, where the ambulette waits. My anxiety rises. Jim will have to push the chair over the curb. Ernest comments on the terrible design—does it even meet the American Disability Act standards? My head bobbles like a trapped weasel. Jim pushes me over the curb. The jolt is tolerable. Ernest gives me a hug. Zoe is behind the ambulette's wheel. Jim instructs her how to lower the platform. He pushes me into position. Zoe joins Jim.

"Keep your elbows inside your chair," Jim instructs. "It's going to be close . . ."

"I think we'd better transfer her," Zoe says.

"I have to be in a wheelchair," I say, frightened that I'll be put on a side-riding bench like the one I rode in to the hospital after my kindergarten boyfriend threw me against the cement-sided sandbox. I think if my father had been home, he would have cleansed my wounds with hot water and iodine and sent me back to school.

"This will work, Zoe," Jim says. "It'll be tight. But it will work. Okay, upsy-daisy."

I feel the platform's rise and someone pushes my wheelchair into tracks on the ambulette's floor.

"Attach her in eight points," Jim barks at Zoe. To me he says, "She's not my usual partner. She's not certified yet."

Zoe is bolting me in on eight sides like I am a spider caught in my own web.

"You're very mechanical, Zoe," I say, dazed by her speed.

"I've had a lot of experience," she says. "Six years."

"But you're not certified?" I ask.

"Paperwork's been delayed," she says. "I got back from Iraq sooner than expected."

"Iraq must have been hard," I say with sympathy.

"I loved it. I liked the work and I liked how much time I had just to hang out."

"Let's go, Zoe," Jim barks louder. He's in the passenger seat. "We haven't got all day."

Zoe undoes my bolts, I keep my elbows close, and ride the platform to the entrance to Dr. Girard's office building. Here there is no curb. Here there is a "Push Here" button—at wheelchair height—to open the wide double-doors into the lobby. Here there is an effervescent, smiling volunteer in a blue vest, acting as if she is the designated greeter at a wedding. Here the elevator's doors are wide. Ernest is here, too.

"Will you sign here, please?" Jim says to the office administrator sitting behind the desk. He hands her a clipboard. "Oh—and the time, too."

"Jim has to document when and where we delivered you," Zoe explains.

"Call us when you're ready to be picked up," Jim says. "Give us about fifteen minutes lead time."

"You'll be the ones to pick me up, right?" I ask. My anxiety is rising. I have learned to trust these two—but would I trust some other two?

Zoe nods her yes, and the two of them scamper off.

Ernest settles into a chair, takes out his Kindle. He's reading Faulkner's first novel, *Soldier's Pay.*

We are waiting. Fifteen minutes pass.

"Is there a lady's room?" I ask the stylish brunette behind the Help Desk.

"Through the door," she says, pointing to the regular size doorway to her left. She notes my wheelchair and says, "Or you can go to the public one near the elevators. It has easy access."

Ernest pushes my chair to the public restrooms and pushes the automatic opening button for the women's room. It has three stalls. Two of them are occupied.

"No family restroom," I say. "I guess we'd better go back to Dr. Girard's office."

I hold my elbows close to my body and Ernest manages to just fit the wheelchair through the doorway. The bathroom has a similar small doorway and no automatic buttons to keep it open. Ernest pushes the chair with one hand and holds the door open with his butt.

"This is exactly what I was afraid of," I say, near tears. The toilet is too low, there are no safety handles, and my Kegel exercises are about to fail me. If the foot-surgeon's ADA bathroom is so difficult for me in a wheelchair, I can hardly imagine the problems in *public* ADA bathrooms, starting with getting into the damn things and holding it together until the one large wheelchair-accessible stall, always at the end of the row of stalls, is vacated by the mother and her baby, diapers changed.

"Here," Ernest says pulling down my pants and holding me up while I precariously stand on my one good foot, bare butt in the air over the bowl. "Pretend you're a man."

On the wall behind the check-in desk is a silver metal sculpture, disjointed with ragged edges. It must be five feet tall and four feet wide, scalpels and scythe blades jagging out in all directions. For the next fifteen minutes I try not to look at it. Then I see a helpful sign: If you are waiting more than fifteen minutes let the desk know. Ernest lets them know.

"Laurel Richardson," a nurse in pink scrubs is calling my name. "Follow me," she says, sprinting toward the inner-sanctum, a room set up with perhaps a dozen hospital beds with white curtains between them.

"Hi. Laurel?" A young man in white scrubs is standing by my wheelchair. "Sorry you had to wait. The paperwork didn't come through. I'm Stuart. I'll be taking your bandages off." He asks me about my foot, my doctor, my rehab facility. "Stretch out on the bed," he says. "This won't hurt." He unwraps my wrappings; my foot and leg are swollen; my skin is flaking. There is no pain. "Your incision looks great," he comments.

Ernest looks. "Not even four inches," he says. "And not inflamed."

"We need to get an X-ray to see about your healing," Stuart says, wheeling me out. "You can wait here," he says to Ernest.

"Watch my purse," I say, like there's something of value in it.

"Step on the platform," says a large African American man who looks like a defensive end and sounds like a television voice-over. "Put your weight on it."

"But I am not supposed to," I whine. Is it my destiny to undo my surgery here?

"It's okay... You'll be okay." He sounds soothing.

"I'm okay?"

"All done," he says. "You did fine. I'll wheel you back to Stuart."

"Sit on the bed," Stuart says. "Dr. Girard will be here soon."

I can hear Dr. Girard's French-Canadian accent a few curtains away. The poor patient he's talking to sounds miserable. So much for privacy. I ask Ernest to hand me my purse, which I rumple through until I find my notebook with my list of valuable questions for the doctor. One should always write the questions down and have them right there in your hand when the doc arrives, for you never know how fast he'll come and go…

"Your X-rays look good, Laurel," Dr. Girard says, unceremoniously parting my white sheet like a … well, like a surgeon. He is attended by the smiling nurse in pink scrubs. He looks at my incision. "Perfect healing… It couldn't be any better… Stuart will fit your cast and I'll see you in two weeks… Well, Dr. Tucker will. Nice seeing you again, Ernest…" Dr. Girard begins dictating into the recorder around his neck.

"I have some questions," I say.

"Shoot away."

I open my paper and try to read my writing. "Let's see. The therapist wants to know exactly how much weight I can put on my foot and when."

"Let pain be the guide."

"No. She wants a specific prescription."

"Twenty-five percent weight—then fifty percent—then 100 percent weight… gradual increments as pain permits." His nurse writes the prescription.

"When can I check out of the Bellemont?"

 "I can't catch her if she falls," Ernest says.

"Not until you are 100% weight bearing," Dr. Girard says, "at least two more weeks… Any other questions?"

"How are you doing after the surgery on your own torn ankle tendon?"

Dr. Girard lifts his pants leg. He is wearing a small brace and a regular shoe. He smiles as he saunters off. Come and gone.

Stuart re-arrives with a pot of goo and asks me to step into it at full weight.

"But Dr. Girard said I shouldn't do one-hundred per cent yet!" I protest.

"It'll be okay this once. I am making a mold of your foot."

I look pleadingly at Ernest, but he is deep into his Kindle.

"Ernest," Stuart says, "You might want to clean off Laurel's foot with this towel."

"Be careful," I say. I could burst out into tears any second. Contradictory directions, unpaid—untrained—labor—Ernest. "Where's the nurse?"

"It's okay. I've got it," Ernest says, and I am relieved because I trust *my* Ernest more than a nurse in pink scrubs.

Stuart returns and puts a long white silky stocking on my leg, and then begins wrapping it. He hands me a key ring of color chips as if I am in a paint store. I chose the dark blue casting tape. It reminds me of my kitchen walls and my upstairs hallway, deep charcoal blue. They in turn remind me of my favorite crayon color of all time—Prussian Blue.

"Good choice," says Ernest. "It won't show the dirt."

"But people won't be able to sign it," I say, having buyer's remorse already, remembering the popularity my arm cast conferred on me when I was six with a broken arm. Kids would ask me if they could sign it. I could have chosen to deny them that exotic experience. I never did.

"I can get a silver Sharpie," Ernest says. "That'll work."

Stuart submerges the blue fiberglass casting tape into a bucket of warm water, and starts wrapping my foot. The non-tacky resin molds to my foot and leg. I am familiar with the technique from book-making and repairing.

"My toes are sticking out," I say.

"We want them to be able to move," Stuart says.

"They are cold."

"You can get a toe-cozy."

"Will I itch under the cast?" I remember my broken arm when I was six, and the horrid itching that I could not scratch.

"No."

"Will my skin peel off?" I remember that happening when I was six and my cast was removed. My arm looked like a mottled lobster claw.

"No. You'll be fine."

"Follow me." The nurse has arrived and leads us to the check-out station.

The director of the Bellemont's therapy is at the counter, too. "Johnetta," I say. "Thank you for coming."

"I want to make sure that we have the prescription."

"Here's everything," the stylish brunette says, handing Johnetta my papers.

Johnetta verifies them and puts them in her purse.

"We're going to the Tim Horton's downstairs for lunch," I say. I've been looking forward to their donut holes for two weeks. "May we treat you?"

"No, thank you. I have to get back."

Ernest calls the LifeHealthCare drivers, and we settle into our lunch. Little girl twins at the table next to us are throwing straws at each other. Before we have finished our wraps, Jim and Zoe arrive.

"We were just around the corner," Jim says.

"Take your time," Zoe says.

"I'll go home and get the dogs," Ernest says.

"Take your time," I say. I put myself into the space between wakefulness and sleep, a space I sometimes enter when I feel afraid, like I do now in the ambulette in my new blue cast.

Renee is waiting outside her door and wheels herself into my room after I return.

"Looks like you're getting better," she says pointing to my cast. "I won't." She looks winsome, coquettish.

"I brought you donut holes from Tim Horton's." I hand her the half-dozen uneaten ones.

"Did you hear all the yelling last night?" she asks.

"I must have slept through it. What happened?"

"Your new neighbor—the fat man—got into it with his wife. They were both screaming about something. She kept saying, 'No, you can't have it,'—sex, I guess. The squad took him to the hospital. I think he had a heart attack, maybe. "

I feel sorry for him but I'm mostly glad that I won't be awakened by his television in the wee hours of the morning. I feel small-minded and selfish and ashamed of my feelings. And then I wonder if they were arguing over the remote?

"How's his wife?" I ask.

"She seemed worried—but, hey, maybe *he* likes women without legs? Maybe I can help her out."

When I was in my late twenties and doing research on vocational rehabilitation, I wore the same professional clothes that I wore for teaching. My male able-bodied colleague criticized me for being "too sexy." He said that sexuality was an issue for the wheelchair bound men we were researching, and that I was making it more difficult for them. After that fall from grace, I changed how I presented myself at the research site. I pulled up the collar on my suit jacket, buttoned it up over cotton blouses, never knit shirts, donned brown oxford shoes, wore my glasses, and pulled my long hair into a bun. I changed how I walked and talked and looked at people. I denaturalized myself, defeminized myself, desexualized myself. By so doing, I realize now, that I had desexualized the wheelchair men, as well.

I do not know if my colleague was correct in his assessment of me or the wheelchair men, but it is clear that sexuality is an ongoing issue for my neighbor, Renee. She is young, beautiful, and energetic. Why wouldn't she have sexual desires?

One of my favorite writers, Nancy Mairs, wrote about how her multiple sclerosis affected her sexuality. She wryly suggests that the sociobiologists might be correct in theorizing that only those suited for reproduction are found attractive. Or maybe the sociologists are correct, that we learn to desire that which we have learned to desire. No doctor or health-care provider has ever asked Nancy Mairs, a married woman, about her sex life. They assume the physically disabled have taken themselves out of the sex-market. The culture teaches us to dissociate a misshapen body from sexuality. We don't want to think about Renee and sex. We are surprised that she does. Maybe she won't a year from now, when the voices from the outside become a voice from within, when she might even question the peculiarity of a man wanting a legless woman, might not trust him at all, decide to accept that her days of being lusted after by a *regular* guy are gone. Or maybe she'll watch over and over again an episode of *The Sopranos* where Tony takes on the Russian lady with a missing leg. But in the meantime, the *conspiracy of silence* (I think that is Nancy Mairs' term) about sex and disability sentences many to opprobrium should they raise the possibility as Renee has.

Jingle-jangle.

"Lily, come up and see me," Renee says. "I'm the one who is *sooo* good to you."

"I stopped at CVS," Ernest says. "Here's a silver pen and the toe-cozy." Ernest puts the black fleece toe sock on my foot and secures it with its Velcro strap. He signs my cast. Renee can't reach it.

"So lookie-heah, y'all," Effie Lou says. "Blue. My fav-rit color. Lemme sign it."

"Am I having therapy today?" I ask.

"Shure-nuff. Wanna try your scooter?"

"God, no! Can you just push me in my wheelchair?"

"Shure-nuff."

"Hi Trevor. See my cast?"

"You can put your foot on this ground-pad." Colleen sets me up on the NuStep.

"I'm afraid," I say. Anytime something new is happening to me, I get afraid.

"You'll be okay," she says. "You'll not be putting weight on it. Just getting to know how the ground feels."

"Don't be a wimp," Rhonda says. I think she thinks she's funny.

Randy's sister is on the large mat. She waves to me. I nod.

The German woman, Ilsa, is doing arm exercises with ten-pound weights. She looks like she wants to throw them at Rhonda.

"Do you have your prescription?" Colleen asks me.

"Johnetta has it. Only 25% weight bearing in the beginning."

Colleen helps me off the NuStep onto my wheelchair.

"You're getting your walker, today," Colleen says.

"What?" I say. "So much in one day?"

"You're ready for it," Colleen says. She positions a walker in front of me, raises its height and takes off its wheels. "Stand on your good right foot and pull yourself up with the walker's arms. Effie Lou will help."

"Upsy-Daisy," Effie Lou says. She is standing behind me.

"Now put your left toes on the ground," Colleen says.

"What? Put weight on them?"

"That's the idea."

"How do you know that'll be 25% ?"

"Twenty-seven years of experience. That's how I know."

Gingerly, I put the ball of my foot on the ground. Nothing breaks. Nothing hurts.

"Walk toward me," Colleen says. "Pick the walker up and take a step on the ball of your foot."

"What?"

"You heard me."

"Won't I hurt myself?"

"No, but let pain be your guide."

I walk the five feet between Colleen and Effie Lou—or did I climb Mt. Olympus?

January 18

———

OH
I have toes
and feet and legs.
What a blessing.

I can stand, stretch.
Another blessing.

I can walk,
grow heavy.

Some day
I won't be walking
in this world,

And when that happens,
that will be a blessing,
Too.

"Hi, Laurel." My dog walker, Thelma, is at the door. Her gray hair is in a long braid, pulled over her left shoulder. "Ernest told me you got your walking cast yesterday and that it would be okay to visit today."

"I'm so glad to see you, Thelma," I say. "And thanks again for taking extra care of Bashi and Lily." When I was still in the hospital following surgery with Ernest by my side, Thelma was at the Paps' sides—taking care of all their needs.

"It's hard to believe that they are almost out of their puppyhoods," I say.

"They'll be dogs before you know it," Thelma says. In the past, Thelma has been a dog-handler and breeder. She's written about dog-aging for dog magazines. "They grow up so fast."

"So, about how long are Papillons expected to live?" I ask.

"Small dogs—twelve to fifteen years," Thelma says. "If you walk them and watch their diets. Like, say, the Westminster Best of Show Papillon, Kirby. He lived for sixteen years. But twelve years is the usual."

"Seven dog years to one human year . . . that's let's see," I do two little multiplications on a napkin: $7 \times 12 = 84, 7 \times 15 = 105$. "I'd like to live until I'm one-hundred," I say, surprised that I desire such longevity because I often wake up with a little prayer of gratitude that I am still alive followed by a little prayer of acceptance—*if this be the last day, then my time has been enough*. When we first got Bashi and Lily, I had hoped that I would predecease them, so I wouldn't have to go through the grief of losing them. But now that we've had them for a year, I want to die after they do, so they won't feel abandoned. Having them is like having perpetual children. I vow to make certain the dogs think of Ben and Tami as another set of loving caretakers, and that I'll leave money for them to put in an invisible fence.

"I'd like to live until I'm one-hundred," I repeat.

"Oh, not me!" Thelma says, horrified by the idea. After a dozen years of renal failure, she found a kidney donor two years ago and her life has gone on, fuller but still limited. This year she turned 65. "I'd like to live another decade but that'll be enough."

I am surprised because I have assumed that anyone who has a transplant—kidney, lung, heart—wants to live—well, forever.

"I know what it is like to be actively dying," Thelma says. "I was doing that for a dozen years—body systems closing down, energy levels exhausted, living in fear, losing social contacts. I don't want to go through that again. Once is enough."

I think about my best friend Betty who died at 69. She thought of herself as 'elderly.' When we were in our thirties, we had a 'joint-reading' of our futures.

"Would we be living near each other toward the end of our lives?" we asked.

"No," the fortune teller said. "You won't."

While Betty was still alive we talked nearly every day. "Did you read my horoscope?" she would ask, as her newspaper, the *New York Times,* didn't consider that news fit to print. On her birthday—October 20—I still read "Your Birthday Today Horoscope for the Year," in my local paper. This year, Betty, you're in excellent spirits. How true . . . For you, I do think, dying was a blessing. An emphysema death. Once is enough.

When Father was in his sixties, we had a long talk about death. "I hope to live my three-score and ten," he said. Religiously, he was now a Deist, believing a creative force had set the universe in motion and then left it to its own doing. Perhaps he constructed a God in his own image? There was, he said, life in all things. People, animals, trees, rocks. Heaven is for you to make on earth. No one expected him to outlive Mother, but he did by three years. On his desk was the day's newspaper opened to a story, "Last Zapata Fighter Dies." The story was in error, as my father was in Troop K, 13th Cavalry stationed at Fort Bliss, led by "Black Jack" Pershing who was charged with the pursuit of Zapata. My father's death on that newspaper's day—July 4th, 1972— made the story true. Father had lived three-score and twelve.

His death has been hard for me because it is unresolved. He was writing his memoirs about his life as a criminal attorney in Chicago— Al Capone was one of his clients—and as a political figure in the Republican party—running for state congress, managing Senator Everett Dirksen's state-wide campaign. Father refused to support Richard's Nixon campaign, though, as Father believed that Nixon had ties to the Mafia. The homicide police in Key Biscayne cordoned off Father's condo and moved his body to the morgue before the family arrived. There was not a sheet of paper in the house. Not a "Father's Day" card. Nada. He was probably murdered. We never saw his body. I asked a Chicago lawyer to look into for me. After he looked into it, he said, "Laurel, you have a house and husband in Ohio . . . Leave it be."

January 19

How different my days here in the Bellemont are from the ones I spend at home. When I am at home, I spend most of the daylight hours in front of my computer, writing. Occasionally, I have lunch with friends, do errands, make phone calls, or go to my group activities. But in the Bellemont either my social-life spins at a full tilt—visitors, staff, therapy, phone-calls—or I am alone, meditative and pensive. I like the change.

"Can I sign your cast?" Brooke is back.

"How's your mother doing?" I ask, handing her the silver pen.

"Much better."

"I see you have a cast." Brandon has come in. "Anything I can do for you?"

"How's the large man who was my neighbor doing—the man who played his television too loud and went to the hospital with a heart attack?" I like the little cause-and-effect I've set up. Creating a story that may not be true is a way to find out the truth.

"He's doing much better."

I guess it was true.

"He'll be back this afternoon."

"So soon?"

"It was only heartburn."

Guess it was only partly true. I'm glad about that.

"In a different room? Please?"

"Yes." Brandon says. "Anything else I can do for you?"

"I don't think anyone official has been in to see my neighbor, Renee."

"We're working on that," Brandon says.

"That ugly one!" Renee is in my room. She is wiping tears from her eyes with her fists.

"What about her?"

"She was giving me a bath and she told me I am lucky not to have legs because it would take so much longer to bathe me if I did."

"Ready?" Colleen has come for me.

"Hi, Trevor."

Colleen sets me up on my walker. My bad foot's toes are on the ground. My hands hold the walker's arms. Effie Lou is waiting a few feet away with a large yellow balloon. Effie Lou and I are going to play volley-balloon, again. I will have to let go of my right hand to play but I won't have the benefit of standing between stationary parallel bars. Effie Lou serves the balloon to me, and I pounce on it with my famous tip shot. A right hand smash!

"Don't hit it so hard," Effie Lou scolds scrambling to retrieve the ball from the large mat area. She serves again. I modify my return now, pretending that Effie Lou and I are on the same team which I guess we are.

"I like playing games at rehab!" I say. "Why don't we play more games? Why does it just have to be exercise? I am ready to reorganize the rehab profession into one that is sports minded, play-oriented, rather than medically framed. Doesn't that make sense? Particularly for the younger ones and the Wounded Warriors?

"I'll walk you on back," Effie Lou says to me.

"How's it going, Effie Lou?" I ask.

"Got me an interview fer the home-health job I tol' you 'bout. Give me more work-time choice."

I hope she doesn't leave before I do!

"Hi, Trevor." I say as we pass him by. He looks asleep.

"Tony's son A. J. has come to live with us," Effie Lou continues. "We've served his ma papers for chil' abuse and chil' endangimint. She's goin' go bee-zerk. We got a keep-away ordeh. No contact. No phone. No drivin' past. No followin' me. "

"How's A. J. doing?" I ask

"Caint get him up for his school bus. So, I git to drive him…jes what I need."

"Is he a good student?"

"Uh-uh. He's a good artist, though. He draws cartoons. I'm gonna get him some real art stuff. Where's a good place?"

"Blick's or Michael's or JoAnne's."

"I kin git him some paper and some cartoon-drawin' books." Effie Lou looks happy.

"Yap, yap."

"Yap, yap, yap."

"Kin I borrow Lily?" Effie Lou asks.

"Sure."

"I'm bringin' her to the long-term ward."

"Yap-yap-yapity-yap-yap-yap!"

"It's okay, Bashi. Lily will be back."

"Hi, Laurel." My friend Jo Dickinson is at the door. Jo is eighty years old, a dancer in her younger years, and now an artist drawn to collage. Her collages move in space, as her body once did. Both Ernest and I had taken creative dance with Jo some forty-five years ago when she taught at the Whetstone Recreational Center. She has come back into my life recently when I signed up for her Artist's Way class. A few weeks into the class, Jo fell, broke her hip, and spent six-weeks in a re-hab facility. I took on facilitating the Artist's Way group.

While she was being rehabilitated, she and her husband decided it was time to let go of the family multi-storied house. He located a condo with mature trees, a swimming pool, and space for both of their art studios. Jo only saw pictures of the condo. She approved. Their house sold immediately to a young family, about which Jo was delighted. "Time for the next generations," she said. John packed up the fifty plus years of "things," and Jo was grateful for the possibility of new adventures.

My visit to her while she was in the rehab was the first time she and I had a "one-on-one." We clicked. Now, she is visiting me—"one-on-one."

"You might enjoy looking at the pictures in this book of contemporary American art," she says, setting the book down next to the violets. "Oh, those flowers! When I was a little girl growing up on the farm, I would take a bit of the newspaper we had for the outhouse, pick dandelions, wrap their stems, knock on a neighbor's door and offer her the corsage. What I loved was the smile she would give me. How surprised she was." Jo *arm-dances* the story.

"When I was a little girl," I say, "we lived in the city. One year my father planted sunflowers at the edge of our yard by the alley. They grew tall and thick and scary and I got lost in them. I yelled and cried and screamed until my mother rescued me."

Jo reminds me of my sister, physically and emotionally. Like her, Jo is small and agile, makeup-free, wrinkled. Each one has met challenges with a certainty of motion. Jo is a gentle sweet soul, a sweetheart who gets great pleasure from gift-giving. That's how my sister was, too.

Do I remind Jo of anyone?

"So, where's my dog Lily?" Renee is at the door.

"Effie Lou has her," Ernest says.

"She's not gonna *keep* her, is she? I get first dibs."

Jingle-jangle.

"Lily was tur-if-ic." Effie Lou carries her into my room, and puts her on my bed. "I put her on Mistah Klein's chest. He cain't move and he's always cold. He doesn't talk much neither. I feared Lily'd be chewin' up the road but she stayed right up there on hiz chest for ten minutes not bein' held or anythin' cause he cain't move his arms. She jes looked at him with them passionated eyes of hers. He talked—said, 'I feel warm.' 'Lily,' I said to her, 'you are a'ready a therapy dog.'"

"You're doing your clinical rotation," I say, giving Lily a hug.

"Good girl!" Ernest says, petting her haunches.

Bashi love-bites Lily's cheek.

"You're getting a new next door neighbor." Renee wheels herself in.

"Hi-Lilly-Dilly, come to Mama." Ernest puts Lily on Renee's lap.

"Looks like it's a woman," Ernest says going into the hallway.

"Has Brandon been to see you?" I ask Renee.

"No, but I have some good news," Renee says. She brightens up. She looks so pretty. "I am getting fit for prostheses tomorrow!"

"Hi, Mom." Josh sounds tired. "Nice cast."

"Hi, Grandma." Akiva sounds tired, too. "Nice cast color."

"We can only stay a little while," Josh says. "I have a math exam tomorrow."

"How's the class going?" I ask.

"The prof's much better than the last one."

"How're things with you, Akiva?" I ask.

"Much better," he says.

I wait.

"My League of Legends team made it to the finals."

Son and grandson sign my cast, give me hugs, and go off into the night.

"Laurel?" Jamal is at the door. "Sorry, I have to weigh you again." Jamal gets me onto my wheelchair and pushes me to the weighing-machine. "Do you think you can stand on the platform?"

"Not yet," I say.

He helps me and my wheel chair onto the platform, subtracts thirty-five pounds for the chair and says, "You've lost weight. Everybody gains here. I don't know why."

"Maybe they eat the food," I say.

Jamal returns me to my room and does his little head-down dance, bouncing like a well placed ping-pong ball from corner to corner.

"I think you're supposed to take my vitals, Jamal," I say.

"I was just procrastinating." He takes out his vitals kit, and attaches the blood pressure machine to my arm. "Two-hundred sixty over one-hundred sixty." He grins.

"I don't think so, Jamal. Try it again."

"One hundred twenty over seventy."

"Much better," I say, and then venture, "You don't much like nurse's aide work, do you?"

"It's a job. I don't know what I want to do."

"Have you been to Columbus State to take their vocational preference test?"

"Not yet . . . no . . . I keep putting it off."

"Do it, Jamal. Take the test."

I know Jamal likes to read novels and poetry. I bet he likes to write, too. I wonder if it isn't just procrastination. I wonder if he's fearful of finding out all his preferences.

He ricochets around my room, as if the corners are possibilities—but not ones he's ready to settle upon, yet.

"Call if you need anything, Laurel," he says, leaving.

"Close my door, please."

January 20

Two weeks have passed. I have been cared for by staff, friends, family and four-legged creatures. All of my bodily, emotional, social, and spiritual needs have been met—most without my asking. No one has treated me as if I am bad person; no one has abandoned me. Quite the contrary. I slide into gratitude and awe. My foot is healing. What else is healing?

Ernest has a doctor's appointment this afternoon, no one is scheduled to visit, and I am off the therapy schedule today. I am feeling good, a little adventurous and secure. I decide to venture away from my routine and scooter to the Bellemont's Family Room. I bring nothing to read, so I will be forced into eavesdropping.

I choose a table in the middle of the room where I can see and hear everything. To my left sits an old man. His carved cane is by his side. His jowls and pants sag. Another old man comes in, walking disjointedly as if his hip-joints are not functioning. "Mind if I join you?" he asks Mr. One, who nods his acceptance.

"My wife's been here for two months," says Mr. One.

"Mine came in last night," says Mr. Two. "They're fixing up her room."

"Our son's here. Visiting. I don't think she'll be coming home."

"I hope mine will."

I am a pushover for old men, in the parks, walking dogs, puffing uphill. In cafes, telling stories of finding oil in Ohio hills, cultivating thornless roses, soft-boiling trout. I like their stories just like I liked my grandfather's stories. His stories could be fairy tales, but they were real.

He, himself, saw the gates of the Czar's court open for teams of white horses pulling coaches with gentry in finery, saw them step out of their fine coaches, saw them enter the Palace. He, himself, fixed the clocks that chimed midnight. But, he didn't know about Prince Charming and Cinderella. Only the real people, although he never told me about the horrendous things those real people did to make him leave Russia, his yarmulke on his head, his prized samovar on his back.

"I went to Indiana on a full scholarship in music," Mr. One says. He's in his eighties, soft spoken and handsome, becoming more so as he speaks. "Then I went to Julliard. My professor told me that I had a nice voice and I would find work but that I would never be a star. I called the music union headquarters and asked what percent of their members could make a living off their music. The answer was two percent. Then, I was drafted."

"I was drafted, too," says Mr. Two. His curly hair is dyed black, his face is tanned, and his red Polo shirt is neatly tucked into his khaki Dockers. He has an old man's wiry body.

Mr. One nods and smiles. Mr. Two smiles back. They have connected at a level I can see, but don't know. My Korean War Veteran brother-in-law Paul would fit right in.

"In the army, "Mr. One continues, "I was given a battery of tests. The tests said I was a lot smarter than I thought I was, and that I would be trained in intelligence—decoding. My life got moved into a direction I had never thought of for myself. Work I really enjoyed. Work that let me support my wife and family. I stayed until I retired."

Mr. Two is nearly jumping out of his chair, as he begins talking. "I was an engineering and math major, but I wasn't very good at them. I wasn't ever going to be very good either. The army gave me a series of tests and I found out that my verbal abilities far outshone my math ones. The army trained me into personnel. I found a career I never would have thought of for myself. I've been happy in management positions ever since."

The two old men look at each other and nod. My brother-in-law Paul could be here. Jamal *should* be here.

I am waiting for them to complain about the war, the government, their benefits, the VA, their lives, but they don't. I wait for them to compete and one-up each other. But they don't. Instead they talk about their marriages, children and grandchildren.

The two old men get up, shake hands, and pat each other's shoulders, the way men do who like each other. These infirm old men are beacons of hope for me. If they can deal with what life has done to their bodies, so can I deal with mine.

My brother-in-law Paul is on mind. Perhaps he is getting even weaker. I scooter to my room and call my brother, Barrie, to find out.

"Paul is a miracle," Barrie says. "He's going to dialysis twice a week and has moved back to his apartment. He's weak and sleeps a lot, but his brain and spirits are good."

"That's great news," I say.

"I don't think so... Our sister could have been here, alive, if Paul had paid attention to her... I don't like his nurse... No one likes her... Everyone thinks he's going to change his will and make her the beneficiary... Maybe give her the power-of-attorney, too."

This is the first time my brother has expressed anger at Paul. Did the anger I let go of find its way to Shreveport, to Barrie's heart? If so, is it helping him to process his grief over our sister's death?

"Have you heard from Cousin Barbara?" I ask.

"She did call. She thought Paul was dying. I hadn't talked to her in over forty-years. Maybe fifty."

"The last time we talked," I say, "she said that father was a womanizer at Camp, and that all the women avoided him."

"No!" My brother has the annoyance in his voice that I remember from my childhood, when he would say no to me, disgusted by the stupidity of my question. "Father was a very handsome man and it was another time—another era—he was expected to flirt with the women. He was doing what was expected of him and they loved it. He was a great dancer. He could have been in a Fitzgerald novel. He was charming, debonair. A lady's man, but he loved his wife and his family. "

Much of what Barrie is saying could also describe Barrie and my son, Josh. Maybe they have a flirt gene.

"Do you remember Cousin Margaret?" I ask.

"That little liar. She lied all the time. She said I set the attic on fire—she was the one playing with the matches. Nobody ever liked her. Not even her family. Especially not her family—they had to live with her—except when she lived with us for awhile."

I find it impossible to believe that my father would have "put his hands" under Margaret's dress—his eleven-year old niece. I know disbelief is common in families; denial of wrongdoing not only protects the powerful family member, but allows the family routines to continue. Ernest wrote a book about this.

"Innocent until proven guilty," was one of my father's mantras. Everyone has a right to be defended was the element of the law that attracted my father into becoming a criminal-defense lawyer, specializing in jury trials, none of which he lost. I wanted to follow in his footsteps, but he nixed it, saying, "Legal cases are decided in Berghoff's Men's Only Bar." Back then, that was true. Nevertheless, Dad, let me indulge my lawyerly-self by making your case . . .

"Dad, I have your photo albums from high school and from your years in the cavalry," I look at an imagined jury in an imagined courtroom. "In the albums there are galleries of women . . . some classy, some looking like camp-followers . . . Many photos are lovingly inscribed to you."

"Yes, that's true." Father's imagined voice confirms. "Your mother didn't like those albums, so I kept them in the bottom drawer of my dresser." I imagine catching the eye of the jury foreman who is imagining all those beauteous women wanting him.

"I know, Dad, about the albums because I rummaged through that drawer when I was a kid." The jury gasps. "The only suspicious thing I found was a cryptic pencil . . . I didn't know what it was for."

"*Styptic* pencil." Father laughs. The men in the jury join in the laughter. "It's for closing nicks after shaving."

"Quiet in the courtroom!" orders the judge.

I pause and make certain all jury members are listening. "I didn't see any pictures of children—or women looking like children."

"What in the world are you talking about, Laurel?" He looks innocent.

"Nothing, Dad . . . nothing."

But, I will continue to practice my attorneyship by reconstructing the supposed scene of the crime. It is late August. Father and eleven-year-old Cousin Margaret are in our five horsepower motor boat on the largest and deepest lake in Wisconsin. Lake Bluestone. Margaret is captaining, but the boat is in danger of capsizing. Father takes over and holds her to prevent her falling out. (He has done that for me, because once I did fall out.) She is wearing a bathing suit. Not a skirt. No child at camp ever wore skirts. Defense rests. Did I do a good job, Dad?

Poor Cousin Margaret. Her four older sisters looked like sisters— blond, short, athletic, green-eyed. Margaret was dark, tall, clumsy, brown-eyed. Her sisters were gymnasts. Margaret played the oboe. Her sisters married their school sweethearts. She married her oboe teacher. Her sisters had many children. Margaret's one child died during its birth. Fifty years have passed since I have seen Cousin Margaret.

Diana and Erica—two members of my memoir-writing group are at my door. The group meets twice a month and has done so for a dozen years. At this meeting there are only the three of us. They've brought lunch from the Chinese Wok.

"Ready to chow down?" Diana asks. Diana helps non-profits raise money from populations that are not culturally accustomed to philanthropy. She's written The Book on it.

"*Chow down.*" I repeat. "That sounds like a Chinese restaurant or a police dog-in-trouble."

"How're you doing?" Erica asks, laughing at my little word-play. She is from England, empathetic and witty. She's worked at Chemical Abstracts, volunteers at hospice, and has completed her MFA in non-fiction. One of her close friends had been in the Bellemont.

"This is hard for you, isn't it, Erica?" I say.
"It brings back sad memories," she says.
"And how's coming here for you, Diana?"
"I find it all fascinating!"

"We brought you some Japanese noodles for dinner," Tami says.
"How're you doing?" Ben asks.
We three chat. Dine on noodles and sip diet Dr. Pepper. They sign my cast, Ben with his odd upside-down left-handed signature and Tami with her perfect Palmer method one. I rejoice that these two found each other. They met in a Holiday Inn hot-tub. Ben belonged to the hotel's health club and was relaxing after his work-out. Tami was celebrating her divorce with her nine-year old daughter, Shana. They made plans to meet the next week-end in Northridge Mall. Ben waited at the east entrance, Tami and Shana at the west one. After an hour of waiting, each one decided they had been stood up and walked toward the Mall's midway fountain, where they threw in coins, made wishes, and met-up. They've been together ever since. Ernest says it's the Universe looking out for them.

CHECK HALL 100 EXIT CHECK HALL 100 EXIT CHECK HALL 100 EXIT RRRRRRRRIIIIINNNNNNGGGGGG RRRRRRRRIIIIINNNNNNGGGGGG

Kiss Me... Kiss Me...

January 21

I am on my scooter on the way to therapy. My new neighbor's door is open and I peek in. "Hello," I say, "I'm your next-door neighbor, Laurel."

"I'm Edna. Glad to meet you." A sweet croaky mid-Ohio accent. Edna is wearing a silky flowered nightgown and matching robe. Her silver hair is in a pixie cut, her nails are manicured, and she is sitting-up in her bed, surrounded by stuffed bears. She is thin as a fairy's wand. "I don't have my make-up on yet," she says. "I hope you don't mind how I look." She winks. "I'm not sure I've been seen without my blush for seventy years."

Make-up (like hair-coloring) is one of the things I put off until I was in my fifties. Only then, upon looking in the mirror, did my father's approval of my naked-face teen-age beauty—"Why gild the lily?"—no longer seem applicable. On my aging lily-face I could see brown spots with light colored edges, wrinkles, and crinkles, "assorted image of death and blight..." Clinique tinted moisturizer, pink blush, a little concealer here and there, and the magic of mascara. Now, in my seventies, I only make-up my face for special occasions, and I still love it when people tell me that I am beautiful.

In my mind's eye is the movie, *The Enchanted Cottage*. I saw it when I was about eight years old. Rather than show his face, a disfigured soldier retires to a seaside cottage where a very plain-looking woman housekeeper takes care of him. As the loving relationship between them develops, he becomes as handsome as Robert Young and she becomes as beautiful as Dorothy McGuire. The audience sees that transformation as well, although it does not really happen. Their flawed appearances reappear if they leave the isolation of the Enchanted Cottage. The upfront cultural messages—"Beauty is in the eye of the Beholder" and "Love Conquers All"—were etched into my brain. But there was a hidden, more insidious message etched deeper in my brain: Being beautiful is superior to being plain.

I remember the Greek story about the artist Zeuxis. He lined up the most beautiful women in Crotona as potential models for the most beautiful of all, Helen of Troy. He selected body-parts and facial features from five different women as no single mortal woman was beautiful enough to represent the Ideal. It must have been a blessing for the Greek women, as none of them were expected to attain the Ideal.

But jump into the modern world. Television, Barbie, celebrity magazines, and advertisements tout a new norm, the perfect size 2 of, say, a Heidi Klum, and the perfect facial symmetry of, say, a Heidi Klum. Forty billion dollars in America are spent annually on diet products. Over ten billion on cosmetic surgery—eyelids, noses, chins, cheeks, necks, breasts. Another six billion on cosmetics and about five billion more on self-help books.

Many authors (notably Naomi Wolf) have critiqued the beauty industry in America that capitalizes on the cultural idea that every woman should be as beautiful as she possibly can. Get on this diet plan, take this weight-suppression pill, apply this pore concealer, buy, buy, buy…apply, apply, apply…buy, buy, buy…Pulchronomic research finds that women feel better if they look good to themselves in the mirror. Better-looking women earn more than their less pulchritudinous sisters. Males, too, are part of the beauty boom. About 15% of facelifts are on men, and they get about 6% of breast-reduction surgeries. The better they look, the more money they make even in occupations for which looks should not matter, like professorships and football teams.

So deeply is the insidious message of *The Enchanted Cottage* woven into the warp and weft of our society that I doubt anyone can grow old or become impaired/physically disabled without feeling stung.

"Shall I get your cosmetics bag for you?" I ask Edna. The artist Zeuxis is said to have laughed himself to death when an old woman asked him to paint her as the model for Aphrodite. I am not laughing at Edna. Instead, I wink at her. How intimate we are already.

"Why aren't you the nicest!" Edna says. "It's on the table."

A dozen blue irises are in a crystal vase in the middle of her table. "What beautiful flowers," I say.

"It's my birthday month flower—February. Lord knows I hope I'm not here until then! George always gets me Irises." She touches her wedding-ring. "Why you'd think Iris was my name." She makes *woo-woo* eyes at me.

"So, Edna, how're you doing?" I ask, handing her a cosmetic bag, printed with yellow irises. It sounds like a forward question, but not too forward because we are already acting like friends. I'm in her bedroom; she's not dressed.

"Why, can you believe it?"

"What?"

"Lord Almighty, I was in my aerobics class at City Workout and I fell and broke my hip."

"City Workout at Graceland?" I ask. My son Ben had belonged there. I am embarrassed as soon as I ask the question, because I am focusing on my family, rather than her broken bone.

"Why, forever more, no!" Edna puckers her lips. Graceland , the first shopping center ever in Columbus lacks caché. Discount specialty stores abound. High Street buses park there. Immigrant Somalians and registered sex-offenders flank the mall's north side.

"Which City Workout?" I ask.

"I go to the one in Upper Arlington. It's near my home." Edna takes her out her hand mirror.

When I first moved to the Columbus area in 1964, the realtor recommended by the math department eagerly showed me Upper Arlington because its restrictive covenant did not allow sales to Negroes or Jews. When I told him I couldn't live there because I was Jewish, he was apologetic, but only, I think, so he wouldn't lose a potential sale. For many years later, I felt uncomfortable with people who lived there— who had chosen to live there, signed the covenant. I was suspicious of university faculty who chose it, they said, "for the schools," which meant schools unintegrated across race or class lines. I did a demographic mapping of where the university's administrators chose to live. It was as enlightening as it was disheartening.

"I go to MacConnell Health Club," I tell Edna. "Or did until I tore my ankle tendon and couldn't do any of the exercises."

"Oh, dearie me. That must be so painful."

"Not too bad, Edna. How about you?" An opportunity to be the good listener I think of myself as being.

"Why, can you believe how fast they get you up and moving? Only a day since my surgery, and Good Lord, tomorrow I'll be starting physical therapy."

"Oh, so there you are, Laurel." Colleen is at Edna's door. "I'm ready for you."

"Hi, Trevor."

"Hi—Hi—Hi."

"About how many steps do you have at home?" Colleen asks. She arches and contracts her back, like the yoga cat/dog posture.

"Three to get into the house. They're new. Concrete. And upstairs to my bedroom about twenty or so and to the basement—television and laundry and cat boxes—about a dozen."

Colleen and I face a wooden mock-up of a stair-case. There are six wide stairs and banisters on each side.

"My stairs are much narrower," I say. "And the distance between the stairs is much greater and there's only one banister and it is round and—"

"Time for you to get some practice then in climbing stairs," Colleen says. "The rule is 'up with the good, down with the bad.' So hold onto the banister and step up with your good right foot."

"Like this?" I ask, as I grasp the banister and use my arm muscles to pull me up onto my right foot."

"Good," Colleen says. "Now bring your left foot up onto the same step. Put only 25% of your weight on it."

"Like this?" I ask. If I didn't already trust Colleen, I would not be able to do it. I fear I'll tear open my wound or stumble and fall and break a hip or a chip a tooth or—

Colleen interrupts my mental catastrophizing. "Good job, Laurel! Now, take a breath. Ready to start down?"

"No!"

"You'll be okay. I've got your back. Put your bad foot down. Down with the bad. Down onto the ball of your foot … down with the bad."

"Down with bad," I whisper as I step backwards off the step.

"Great! Now bring your good foot down to the same stair."

If I could magnetize myself to the banister, I would. This is scary.

"Good job! Now let's try it again. Up with the good."

"I'll walk her on back," Effie Lou says. She looks like she's been crying. "I'll take her scooter while she works on her walker." We slowly travel together down the long corridor, past the Family Room, past Trevor, past Edna's room, me picking up the walker taking a baby-step with my good foot inside the walker's perimeter and bringing my bad foot up to match it, starting again, baby-step by baby-step. Effie Lou's trembling.

"Bad night, Effie Lou?" I ask.

"Yep. Worsest."

I wait.

She wipes her nose with her sleeve.

I wait.

"Last night, Tony said to me, 'Fuckin' you makes me feel like a prostitute.'"

Jingle-jangle.

"Oh, Ernest," I say, "poor Effie Lou." And I tell him the story.

"That marriage is over," Ernest says. "How can she ever get past that?"

Knock-knock.

"Effie Lou? Come in."

"Kin I borrow Lily for a bit?" she asks.

Knock-knock.

"Come on in, Effie Lou."

"Lily gave me the sweetest kisses," she says, giving Lily a kiss right between her ears.

Ernest wheels me into the corridor with Bashi and Lily on my lap.

"Hi, Edna," I say. Her door is open.

"Come on in and chat a bit." Edna's wearing a iris-colored silk bed-jacket. She has her make-up on, blue-black mascara, pale lavender eye shadow, smudges of concealer on her cheeks. "Are those darling Papillons yours?" she asks.

"Yes. Lily and Bashi."

"We had two AKC King Charles Spaniels—Prince and Princess—they lived 'til they were oldsters. That was years ago. They died within days of each other. Just like spouses do. Well, men do if their wife goes to the Lord first. Have you met my husband, George?" George looks sporty and dapper in his lavender golf shirt and Mephisto loafers. I recognize the brand because Ernest has a similar pair I bought for him years ago, deeply discounted at Filene's Basement. I bet George didn't get his loafers at Filene's.

"Hi, George," I say. "I saw you in the Family Room talking about your World War II experiences."

"Very nice to meet you," George says, standing up. "Very nice."

"Meet my husband, Ernest."

"Thanks for your service, George," Ernest says. The two men shake hands.

"Will you bring the Papillons over tomorrow?" Edna asks.

"I'll clean 'em up just for you," Ernest says.

Ernest wheels me to the exit. He carries the dogs out the door, and I wheel myself back. I am looking forward to a quiet Saturday night in my own private room with a view of the moon, and with nothing I have to do for or with anybody. But then I see Renee's father standing near the nurses' station, his head hung low.

"Hi," I say. "I'm Renee's neighbor, Laurel. We met a bit ago."

"Yes, the dog lady. Thank you for being a friend for Renee." He brushes his cheek. He is so thin and gray, gray everywhere—hair, eyebrows, skin tone, pants, shoes. It is hard for me to imagine he was once a commander of troops, a survivor of battles on foreign shores, a military husband and father—stuff that Renee's told me about him. Easy to see why he would choose to retire back to the town where grew up. I am thinking about him this way because I can't get my mind around what it would be like to see one of my children legless. And I don't want to get my mind around it. I don't want that image in my head. So, I refocus on Renee and say, "How hard it must be to see your daughter."

"Yes and she's so demanding—always was, but it is worse now. She wants us to come every day and stay all day. We live in Logan—that's over a ninety-minute drive each way. Her mother has osteoarthritis so she can't come that often."

"What a lot of responsibility for you, then."

"Yeah, both my wife and my daughter. And I'm not young, you know. I'm 88. Too old for all this."

I nod and wait. I sense there is more.

"Renee keeps thinking she can return to her two-story house. She's being completely unrealistic. She's always been headstrong. She won't listen to anyone."

"It is so hard," I say.

Renee's father looks down at me in my wheelchair. Perhaps I look vulnerable and non-threatening. Plus, I am a stranger—we are strangers in a hallway, passing strangers. His body seems to sustain a punch in his gut, as he continues talking. "We lost our older daughter suddenly from pancreatic cancer. I thought that was the worst thing I could experience. The sudden death of Donna, only in the hospital less than a week—moved from the hospital to hospice, and then she died. My wife hasn't recovered and now it's Renee. I think this is worse… Renee'd be happier dead."

And so would you?

I ask myself, And so would I? No, I think my arms would embrace life. I hope they would.

January 22
——————

"Special breakfast, Laurel." Brooke glides in, like a mermaid. "Cranberry juice, bananas, French Toast, cinnamon and sugar on the side. And the Sunday paper. Plus your rice milk and cereal." Brooke's blond hair looks like tendrils from the sea, zigging and zagging. Seeing her jubilance is like witnessing a rising tide.

"Have you been swimming this morning?" I ask her.

"Just a late start getting my hair washed."

"Did you have a fun Saturday night?"

She grins, and flips her left hand at me. On her ring finger is a diamond ring.

"Congratulations!" I say, then remember manners taught me nearly seventy years ago at White Gloves and Bow-Ties Etiquette School. Regarding nuptials, one says "Congratulations" to the man, and "Best Wishes" to the woman. Was this an incantation of reality? Was the man a hunter who had caught his prey? Did the woman need "best wishes" to have a happily married life? Waiting in the bridal room before my marriage to my now ex-husband, my mother said something like, "You have to put up with what you have to put up with." She put up with a philandering husband, my father. Like other men of his social-class and generation, he had a mistress. I met her once.

"We've moved the wedding date up. Mom wants to be there, so it'll be before her next brain surgery. I want her there." Brooke's blue eyes look bluer, wetter now with tears. She raises her eyes to the heavens.

"Hi, Trevor. It's me. Laurel. I'm using my walker."

"Oh, hi. Is this the way out?"

"You need to wait here, Trevor."

"Wait here?"

"Yes."
"Okay."

"Where's Effie Lou?" I ask when I reach the Therapy Room.

"She's taking the day off," Rhonda says. She rolls her eyes and draws air circles with her index finger pointing to her brain.

"I'm Melissa, your subbing occupational therapist today." Melissa is a pregnant no-nonsense brunette. She flips through my chart. "Let's see. You are to learn to bathe yourself today."

"I've been sponge-bathing myself since I got here," I say, a little indignantly. Does she think I'm a dud? I am unabashedly suspicious of new helpers. She hasn't done anything wrong *yet*. I smile my apology to Melissa.

"Time to take a real bath," she says. "Let's see. You will use the DryPro cast cover on your cast. Hmm? Has anyone seen Laurel's cast cover?"

"She can just use a Glad garbage bag, like the others do," Rhonda shouts from her desk. She's doing toe-raises.

"I'm not going to wrap my cast in a Glad bag," I announce. "Dr. Girard ordered the DryPro for a reason." I love naming authority figures, dropping them in just when I need them to bolster my case, disguise my orneriness. "I am not going to risk getting my cast wet."

"You go, girl," the broken-hipped Edna is doing arm exercises. Her shirt is gold and black, the Upper Arlington High School colors.

"Thanks, Edna."

"You go, girl? Huh?" Violet is popping her beads. "Who's calling *me* 'girl'? HUH?"

Ilsa the German woman shadow boxes.

An elderly man in a wheelchair looks hopeful—a therapy-room brawl maybe?

Melissa searches a back closet and returns with a plastic bag that holds my specially ordered periwinkle blue latex cast cover, guaranteed to be waterproof. "Not sure how this works," Melissa half whispers, as she reads the directions. "Step one: Stretch the cast cover so it completely covers the cast plus an additional inch with the top smooth against the skin."

"It's too tight!" I say. "Stop it!"

"Complain—complain—complain." Rhonda says between lunges.

"It is too tight," Melissa says. "Let's see. Oh, it says to trim the top." She cuts off an inch of latex. "There, is that better?"

"Much better."

"Step Two: Pump out the air with the attached hand-held bulb until the DryPro is tight to the cast and wrinkled. Like this, I guess." Melissa pumps away. "A vacuum seal!"

Melissa opens the door to the instructional-use-only bathroom. "The bath tub," she tells me," is equipped with a hand-held shower head and a swivel seat sliding transfer bench with backrest. You see. State of the art. You might not be able to afford to buy one of these for your home, though." Then why am I being instructed on it? And if an upper-middle class woman with money in the bank probably won't be able to afford it, who can? I think the apparatus is here for the therapist's convenience, not the patient's... maybe here for show... maybe governmental funds pay for it... top of the line and all that...

"So, get undressed now, and I'll help you get on the seat."

I feel embarrassed and vulnerable. I am in a bathroom that anyone could enter. No sign says *Occupied*. Melissa is a total stranger to me. A voyeur.

She holds my naked body with its bright-blue leg-cover in a standing position and directs me to sit on the bench that is outside the tub.

"Has that bench been antiseptically cleaned?" I ask, not liking the idea of putting my bare butt where other bare butts have gone before me.

"Of course," Melissa says, dismissing my fear-factor. "Now, grab the arm rest for support and lift each leg over the tub wall."

"It's facing the wrong direction," I moan. "The backrest should face the other way so my leg is protected."

"Your leg is protected. You have the DryPro."

"I want that leg to stay out of the tub."

Melissa snarls—not really but sort of—and reorients the backrest and readjusts the hand-held shower head. She leaves me to my lather. I am through with my bath and shivering. There is no call button that I can reach from my swivel. "MELISSA!" I yell.

"Sorry," she says. "I was on the phone. Let's see. We can get this latex DryPro cover off you by just breaking the seal and letting the air back in. I'll help you out of the tub." She hands me a towel and watches me dry-off. How can anyone dry their private parts with a stranger watching? She helps me dress. I am exhausted. I'll never do this again.

"Feel better after your bath?" Rhonda asks. A little mean smirk crosses her face. "You have to show improvement, or you can't stay here."

Trevor's wife—daughter?—is sitting next to his wheelchair.
"Hi, everyone," I say.

Renee is outside my room, waiting for me.
"Can I come in?" she asks, cocking her head. She's been crying.
"What's up?" I ask.
"That mean one—the one from Sierra Leone—was giving me a bath and she said I was lucky I didn't have any legs because then how much longer it would take to bathe me." Renee starts crying.
I don't say *Renee, you already told me that...* instead I say, "Oh, Renee, that's terrible."
"Why would anyone say something like that?" she sniffs. "I've reported her."
Renee returns to her room and closes the door.

I hear the familiar "jingle-jangle," "yap, yap" of my Paps and go into the hallway to greet them.
"Well, he-low Pappy-Doodle-Bugs!" Edna calls. Her door is open. She is in her bed. A "Golden Bear" throw covers her legs. "Come on 'a my bed," Edna half-sings. Ernest puts the dogs on her bed. "C'mon be happy," Edna sings to the dogs. Bashi looks nervously at me. Lily howls like a back-up singer.

"I bet you were a cheerleader in high-school," I say.

"Lordy-Lordy, how'd you guess?"

"And I bet your son played lacrosse for UA high school."

"You are one whiz-kid. But, no. He played soccer! Gotcha!!"

"How'd your therapy go?"

"Aren't we the lucky-ducks to be *here*!"

Lucky to be here? We're lucky to be upper-middle-class white American women with financial means and Medicare, women who have had access to the best doctors, hospitals and rehab facilities in Columbus, women who have learned to eat well and exercise. Being *here this year* is another place and time for our lives of privilege to continue on their beneficent journeys as my insurance company has written me that next year the Bellemont will be terminated from their provider list. I feel grateful that I am here, now.

"Here's my puppies." My Art League friend Randy has come in with Frida and Diego, two long-haired Chihuahuas. They have matching red-checkered bandanas around their necks. They are greeted by our two brave Papillons yapping their heads off. "Are you safe from these intruders? Let us protect you? We are small, but mighty guard dogs!" According to my favorite dog book, Papillons have been bred to be guard dogs from at least the sixteenth century. King Henri III of France, having declared them the official guard dog of the Royal Court, chose three to serve as his personal bodyguards. Henri's favorite was Lilene, an especially small and lovely female. She tried to save his life by barking relentlessly at a man falsely claiming to be a monk. Henri remanded her to another room. Once alone with Henri, the assassin stabbed the monarch. Henri's final words were regret that he had not heeded poor Lilene's warning.

"The Chihuahuas are our friends," I say to Lily and Bashi.

"They're good dogs," Ernest says, reassuringly.

Frida is cowering by Randy's legs. Diego is drinking from the Paps water bowl. His bandana is getting wet. Lily and Bashi are circling the bowl.

"*Yap. Yap. Yap.*"

"BARK. BARK." Diego's talking.

"BARK. BARK." Frida's talking.

"I brought Lily a hot-pink cable-knit sweater that just doesn't fit Frida right," Randy says, opening a plastic bag. "See the cute heart on its backside? Sorry, I don't have one for Bashi."

"That's okay," I say. "Thanks. Can Frida and Diego have some liver treats?"

Did someone say 'treats'?

All four dogs stop their "woofing."

"Sit," I say. And four dogs sit.

"Four good dogs," Ernest says, giving them liver snacks.

"Thanks," Randy says. "And my sister thanks you for your visit."

"I saw her in therapy. On the mat."

"It's not going to work. She's too weak to stand, and they've told her that she's not making progress and will have to leave … and … and … and … and … I'm sorry I have to leave so soon, but I do."

Our Papillons settle on the floor; they look relieved.

Ring-ring. Jean's Sunday call.

"Hi, Mom." Son Josh gives me a cheek-kiss.

"Hi, Grandma." Grandson Akiva does the same.

I like these Sunday predictables.

"Sunday dinner—roast beef, gravy, mashed potatoes, green beans and chocolate cake. Just what you ordered," Vena, the Sierra Leone nurse's aide brings in my tray and sets it on the table. She reaches over my bed and tickles Lily behind her ears. "Should I get another tray for the dogs?"

"They can have my leftovers," I say. "But thanks."

"Come on, Pappies! Let's go do your business," Ernest says, noting Lily going around in circles, sniffing.

Vena looks disappointed as the Paps follow Ernest out the door.

"Where have you been?" I ask Vena. "I haven't seen you in a while."

Vena stares at me. I sense an uncertainty in her look. Does she wonder if Renee told me the bathing story?

"It's nice to see you," I say.

She stares at me again, then speaks. "My car broke down and I didn't have the money to repair it. You can work in America for five years and not have $5,000 saved. You can work all the time and have nothing. It's not like that in Sierra Leone. It's not like how you think about Africa. Oh, poor Africa. No, if you have a little money, you can get very rich. There are a lot of very rich in Sierra Leone … diamonds. You know about diamonds?"

"I do, Vena."

We both wait. I think she's waiting for me to contradict her. I don't.

"So, my car was broken and I had to come on my friend's work schedule. I lost my time in the skilled wing. You are in the skilled wing and I am a state certified nurse's aide." She stares at me again. I feel accused. Of what? Being sort-of-able-bodied? "So, I lost my time in the skilled wing," she repeats. "So, I have to work in the unskilled wings." She empties my waste-basket.

"I'm sorry," I say. "That must be hard."

Vena stares again. There is an unsmilingness in her soul, a festering of anger, an attitude that says *you have no idea, you woman of privilege.* "You gotta change diapers—diapers on fat men—fat women—skinny men—skinny women with bones that break. Change their dirty sheets. Spray their dirty mattresses. Smell their dirtiness. Turn them over. Listen to them yell at you—threaten to kill you—call you Nigger—throw their food at you—spit at you. Hit you—hit you on the head—pull your hair—hit your body—touch you. Try to touch your … and you can't hit back and you have too much to do and the nurses won't help. They tell you to work faster and the families complain about you and you can't quit the job because you need it."

"Oh, Vena. I am so sorry." My inner sociologist comes out. Vena's work experiences in the unskilled wards—bullying, threats of violence, actual violence, sexual harassment, hard unpleasant physical labor, lack of support, and lack of control over her work—are precisely those conditions associated with depression and post traumatic stress disorder. No wonder her soul does not smile. Not only has she experienced traumatic stress disorder, she will continue to re-experience it.

I ask, "Does the management do anything to protect you from violence?"

Her eyes say *Are you crazy?* Her voice says, "Every body is a bed paid for."

"Do they help you deal with the verbal abuse?"

You don't get it, do you? Says the flip of her head.

"I'm going to talk to Brandon about what you've told me," I say.

"Don't tell him it was me!" All her movement stops. She freezes for a second and then her fast breathing becomes audible. She is afraid. "Tell him, I talked about the nice couple in Ward B, who throw good-night kisses to each other . . . kiss me, kiss me . . . they say to each other." But all the kisses in the day or night will not make Vena well and safe, she knows it, her supervisors know it, the management knows it, the owners know it, and now I know it.

Jingle-jangle.

Lily and Bashi sit in front of Vena. Vena picks up Lily, gives her a hug and sets her on my bed.

"Take-care, Vena," I say.

"Call if you need something," she says. She leaves humming *Sweet Silver Bells.*

CHAPTER 10

Down With The Bad, Up With The Good

January 23

"Effie Lou, I am so happy to see you!" I say, after scooting my way to the Therapy Room. "I missed you."

"Ya'll cleaned up nice," she says, handing me five-pound hand weights. "Are your dogs comin'?"

"Soon."

"I got it in mind to get me a little dog. Ah saw one on-line. I'm goin' for it."

"Hi, Laurel." Renee's voice. This is the first time I've seen her in the Therapy Room. She's smiling. She looks fetching. "I'm getting fitted for a prosthesis today."

"That's great."

I'm not sure I would want prostheses.

Renee wheels to the back of the room where a sheet is drawn around her, the p.t., Prem, and a short man in a white jacket

"Ready Laurel to climb two steps today?" Colleen asks. "It's the same as one step—only it's two."

"Ha-ha!"

"And you can try weight-bearing fifty percent."

"How will I know?"

"Go about half way up your foot. Remember—up with the good, down with the bad."

"What happens if I mix 'em up?"

"You can't bend at the ankle when your foot is in a cast. If you go down with your good, you'll go up on your casted leg's toes and they'll slip out from under you and you'll fall… Well, you won't when I'm here, anyway."

This is serious, not just a clever aphorism.

With trepidation, I follow Colleen's instructions. I walk up two steps and down two steps. Mt. Everest here I come!

"Hi Trevor." Trevor looks glum, today.

"Anything I can do for you?" Brandon the business manager has come into my room.

"Maybe get the grunting Corridor Woman to move away from my door?"

"I can do that, or try to. Hearing grunting sounds is one of the major complaints we get from the rehab patients. Anything else?"

"My bed doesn't stay put when I try to transfer to it," I say.

"Let me tell Gunther about it. Anything else?" Brandon is bouncing about my room. I think he wants to hang out for awhile with me. Well, why not?

"So, did you and your wife do anything special this weekend?"

"Oh, I'm not married."

"Oh, I thought you were."

"I'm engaged. My fiancé is not finished with school. She's very busy with her studies, She goes to Bowling Green University and it's a long drive to see her and she has to study."

"What's her major?"

"Elementary education."

Brandon goes on to tell me that they met in junior-high school and have been engaged for four years. They haven't set a date yet for the wedding because he wants to be financially secure and able to provide a down payment on a house in case she wants to start a family right away. His job at the Bellemont is still probationary.

"I hope to find a management position," Brandon says, "in a private continuing-care community that offers care from independent living to hospice. Fewer restrictions, better work conditions, and…" He looks anxious.

"Better morale?" I finish for him.

"Yes." He breathes a sigh of relief. "Yes. That would be better. There's about a 70 percent turnover in nurse's aide staffing at the Belle-mont. We're lower than the national average, though. In some facilities the turnover is 400 percent each year. It's expensive for us to recruit and train new staff and it is not good for the residents having to constantly adjust to new aides. It's much better if the aide knows the likes and needs of each resident rather than expecting the resident to adjust to the new aide. The health of the residents suffer."

"I think mine would, too, if I had a different aide all the time. I've really appreciated the continuity of having Brooke, Jamal, and Vena as my aides."

"It is easier to retain the aides in your wing. Rehab."

"Can't the management do something about staff retention in the long-term wings?" I ask. *The sicker just get sicker.*

"There is this idea to create self-managed work teams to give more autonomy to the aides. The idea is for the aides to take on some of the management of their own work. They would plan the logistics, decide who works what holidays, what shifts, what patients and monitor their service. If they have some control of their work life, morale will improve and turnover will decrease."

"Some corporations and manufacturing firms use that model," I say, feeling proud of my sociological knowledge.

"Yes," Brandon concurs. "And, the efficiency in those corporations actually increased."

"Best be careful, though, Brandon," I say. "You might efficiency yourself out of a management job."

"Not likely, yet. But, this is a for-profit facility," Brandon reminds me. "We are very regulated. Medicaid. We might not be allowed to give much autonomy to our nursing staff."

"Aren't the continuing-care communities regulated?" I ask.

"The private continuing-care communities fall under homeowners laws. This makes it easier to institute changes that benefit staff and residents. Plus, many of the residents in assisted living and nursing components hire private nurses and aides. So everything is easier for everybody."

"My brother-in-law bought into one of those communities. He's in assisted living. He's hired a helper 24/7."

"He's fortunate to have the resources for that." Brandon smiles.

"Yeah," I say. I don't tell him the money is from my sister's portfolio. She started buying blue-chip stocks when she was eighteen.

"The Bellemont's going through some changes in mission," Brandon continues. He looks proud. "We are increasing our percentage of rehabilitation patients. Patients like you are nearly 60% now. Our new equipment in the Therapy Room is one of our selling points. Rehabilitation patients are easier for the staff, that makes retention better. It makes good financial sense to do what we're doing."

How many years has it been since I've had a long conversation with a traditional man?

"Okay, if I take the scooter out?" Gunther asks. "It's pretty crowded in here."

A scooter, wheelchair, walker, DonJoy IceMan, DryPro, round table, four table chairs and a dog's water dish all one side of the room.

"Thanks, Gunther." How important the responsive and capable handy-man Gunther has been to my feelings of safety and being looked-after. He has one of those invisible jobs that we all depend upon. "And thanks again for all you've done."

I ride my wheelchair through Wing B with the moaning, crying, spitting, soiling souls vacant-eyed on wheelchairs, or worse, accusative-eyed, poking fingers in the air toward me, or choking in their beds screaming, "Help me . . . Help me."

"Bingo's going to start," the Activities Director says, flat-voiced.

Bingo is the only supervised group game the higher functioning long-term residents of the Bellemont play, although I hope they still have the wits and will to play other games with each other like "Gotcha," "Yes, but...," "See what you made me do," and other such games people play as thoroughly analyzed by Eric Berne in his book *Games People Play*, popular in their salad days and happily taught by me to my first Sociology 101 class. According to Berne there were three different ways grownups could interact with one another: adult-to-adult; parent-to child; child-to-child. Only adult-to-adult interactions led to mental health.

"There's a place—*here*—for you," the Director says to me in a parental tone of voice. She points to a space at the table.

"I'm going to get my hair washed," I sing-song back in my sweet child voice.

I try to remember when and where I played Bingo and why I don't like the game. I know I did not play at Family Camp because camp was Presbyterian and Bingo was considered a Catholic game. *BINGO!* My Bingo playing happened at Our Lady of Something Catholic Church on Friday nights after the fish-fry, where I, aged 6 or so, would sit in the odiferous basement at a long table with my high-school aged sister Jessica, who was probably charged with my child care. We were with her boyfriend, Paul, and Paul's embarrassingly overweight mother in a dressy-dress, house-slippers for her gout, and noisy false teeth. After endless announcements, during which I snuck peeks at the life-sized Jesus pinned to a cross and the mini-Jesus on a chain resting right in the middle of Paul's mother's chest, the turner would turn the cage with the cubes and the caller would call the winning numbers and I never won. I never once said "Bingo!"

"Aren't you the lady with the Papillons?" A woman who looks like an ermine, all white, slithery and sleek asks. She has a Bingo card upside down in front of her.

I nod.

"Oh, bring them to my room. Do you have a camera? I do. I can take the picture. Room 3937. I can take the picture. I have a camera on my phone. My granddaughter wants to groom Papillons. She took a grooming test and passed. She passed. But PetCorp fired her. I can take a picture. I have a camera."

"Beth, it's time to start the Bingo game," the Director says, turning her Bingo card right side up.

"Can't I have two cards? I can do two cards. I want two cards. Can I have two cards?"

"Here, then." The Director gives Beth a second card.

"See you all later," I say, not intending to. I wheel myself to Mildred's Beauty Salon.

Jingle–jangle.

"Can I borrow Lily?" Brooke glides in. She sets a glass of cranberry juice on my table.

"So let me see now about this bed of yours," Gunther comes in. He and Ernest nod their hellos. Bashi is on the bed. His tail is not wagging.

"It's okay, Bashi. Gunther is a *friend*," I say. Bashi wags his tail. "Friend" is one of his thirty-five words.

Gunther shakes his head. "This bed should be replaced. The wheel-locks are broken. They could move you to another room. . ."

Ernest shudders. I shudder. *No, not that!* I am known for starting out in one hotel room and finding fault with it requiring us to move to another room and maybe even a third one. Ernest doesn't even go into the assigned hotel room nowadays, until I've judged it satisfactory.

". . . or," Gunther continues, "I could rig stoppers for it. The staff couldn't move it, but you'd be safe. Which shall it be?"

"Stoppers, please."

I rest back on the bed and look out my window to the ersatz dog-park. It is a surprisingly warm and sunny day. The smoking lounge is full, and Brooke has wrapped Trevor in several blankets and wheeled him outside. Lily is on his lap. Trevor does not look glum. Diminished man and brave dog—best friends.

"See you later, Darling," Ernest says, scooping up Bashi and Lily in one arm, hugging me with the other. I hear the jingle-jangle as they meander down the corridor to the exit door.

Knock-Knock.

"Come in." It's Dan! Dan is married to Ernest's daughter, Deirdre. He's a big guy, once a wrestler. He bow hunts, primitive camps with his buddies, coaches his daughter's soccer team, co-parents, enjoys life, and affably follows his own moral compass. After seven years of missionary work in Russia, he continues his calling, working long hours at work, home, and his church. I am surprised and delighted that he has come to visit me.

"How're you doin'?" Dan asks, giving me a hug.

"Pretty good. Thanks."

"It's the darndest thing," Dan chuckles, wags his head and slaps his thighs. I know he's about to tell me a real-life story that he sees as a story when others might not.

"What is?" I ask.

"I came in through the awning door and looked for the greeter." He slaps his thighs again. "No one was there." He shakes his head. "So, I walked on in, up to the nurses' station, and I asked what room you were in. The nurse didn't look up at me, she just kept writing, she didn't take a glimpse at me, and said Room 112." Dan is having more fun than a monkey's uncle. "I could have been a mass-murderer! I could have been a hit-man! I could have been from the IRS!"

"So much for privacy and protection," I say. "But Renee, my across the hall neighbor, has top security clearance, so you'd better be who I think you are."

"Did you know I used to work here when I was in high school?"

"Nurses' aide?" I ask, having trouble imagining Dan in that job.

"Nah. Mostly I carried stuff up from the basement."

"I didn't know they had a basement."

"It's kind of creepy." Dan is laughing again.

Another story? No, he's suppressing that one. Probably thinks it is too gory for me to hear.

"Nothing's changed here," he says. "It's kind of creepy that twenty-five years later everything's the same."

"It's been painted. Yes?"

"I don't know. Maybe the same colors."

"How's work going, Dan?" Dan works for a Christian outreach. About a year ago he took on administrating their new outreach in Coshocton County. Raising money is a continuing problem. "We're having an event for our big donors." He shakes his head. "Our big donors are those giving over a thousand dollars in a single year."

With the resources they have, Dan tells me, they provide educational support for middle- and high-school kids at risk, interventions for kids in the juvenile justice system, retreats and community service opportunities. I am moved to become a "big donor"—even though I do not believe in his religion, I do believe in Dan.

"Well, I gotta get back," Dan says, giving me another hug. He has hung-out with me for ninety minutes. This is the first time he and I have spent any extended face-to-face alone time. How remarkable it is to be in the rehab center!

"Do you need anything?" Jamal is at my door.

"Have you been to Columbus State yet for vocational counseling?"

"Not yet."

"What're you reading, Jamal?"

"Ralph Ellison." He looks down, avoiding eye-contact.

"*Invisible Man?*"

"Have you read it?"

"Years ago. What do you think of it?"

"I like that the black narrator doesn't have a name, and that he's living rent-free in the basement of a whites-only building. That's how it used to be. I like reading about how things were. Ellison's telling his autobiography."

Jamal bounces from foot-to-foot.

"Tell me more, if you want."

January 24

"Do you need anything, Miz Laurel?" Vena's voice.

"Can I help you in any way?" Brandon's voice.

"Is everything okay?" The Social Director's voice.

"Do you need anything?" A familiar man's voice.

"How is everything going?" An elderly woman's voice.

"Doing okay, Laurel?" The Admission Director's voice.

"You, Laurel, you feel good?" The beautiful nurse Kiendra's voice.

"Do you need anything?" Brandon's voice again.

"Everything okay?" The Activities Director's voice.

"How's it going, Laurel?" Colleen's voice.

"How y'all?" Effie Lou's voice.

"Any problems? Complaints?" Two unfamiliar voices.

Inquiries about my well-being all day long!

"Renee," I wheel out of my room into hers. "Do you know what is going on?"
"Didn't you hear the commotion last night?" Renee asks.
"No."

"A patient was brought in last night and his wife didn't think they were handling him right or moving quickly enough." Renee looks gleeful to share the gossip. "She started yelling and screaming at the squad guys and she hit one of them and threatened a nurse. Someone called the police who escorted her out of here. She called the state to report this place as derelict, which it is, so, today there's been an unscheduled visit from the state evaluators." Renee's glee runneth over. "The staff are all running around. Now they are paying attention to me. I gave the state a mouthful."

January 25

———

I am in the Bellemont's Family Room. Ernest has gone to the drugstore. The Papillons are sleeping at my feet.

"There's Laurel," the still beautiful Nathalie says, pointing me out to her husband Joseph, a retired OSU English Professor. Nathalie is barely taller than the wheelchair that Joseph is in. She says, "Joseph's had a stroke."

"I see dogs," Joseph announces.

"He's hallucinating," Nathalie whispers over his shoulder. "He does that."

"Yap."

"Oh, he's not." Nathalie reaches down and pets Bashi.

Joseph's voice and bearing always seemed ministerial to me, in the good sense, and his wife always seemed like an angel. They've endured serious illnesses with their children and grandchildren, and I am sorry to see this turn of events in their lives.

"I am still sorry," I say to Joseph "that I never sat-in on your Literary Marriages course. Everyone raved about it."

Joseph smiles and cracks a joke, I think. His speech is slurred.

"It doesn't look good for Joseph," Nathalie whispers.

"There *you* are! I've been looking for you . . . You weren't in your room." Olivia has come in. She's a retired English professor, too. She's had the misfortune of having her life's work on Thackeray badly reviewed by her major literary adversary. This has kept her from promotion to full professor. Over the years she has held various administrative posts in the department and college. Now, she is double-dipping, having been re-hired into the department as a "Human-Relations" administrator. She has gained an inordinate amount of weight. "I've brought you a release form from the English Department—oh, and their get-well wishes. Can you sign the form?"

"Olivia, he can't," Nathalie says. "I have his power-of-attorney but I'll have our son look at the form. Joseph's tired, now. I'm wheeling him back to his room."

"See you later, Nathalie," I say.

"What are *you* doing here?" Olivia notices me.

"Ankle surgery," I say.

"Oh."

"Have they found Bob Larson?"

"Who's Bob Larson?"

"The professor who was in your English Department. He's missing. He has Alzheimer's. There's an alert for him on the news and the highway signs."

"I don't remember him."

I remember that Olivia headed up the "gang of five" who tried to prevent Bob's tenure claiming he sexually harassed undergraduates.

"How's Charlotte Smythe doing?" I ask. Charlotte was a history professor who left on disability and is wheelchair bound. She and Olivia were the strong feminist contingent in their college for two decades. Charlotte was part of the "gang of five."

"I don't know. I don't see her."

"You don't?"

"We're not friends. See you later, Laurel. Oh, how's Ernest?"

I doubt if Olivia hears me say, "Fine."

My mind turns to happier and friendlier times in academia. My first academic appointment was at California State—Los Angeles. Most of my students at Cal State were much older than I, the first in their families to go to college. Most held full-time jobs as blue collar workers. They were eager to learn; I was eager to teach and learn. I taught five different classes a semester and it was the easiest teaching I have ever done. I liked my colleagues, too, and found them intellectually challenging: Franz Adler, a Jew who escaped Germany and worried about anti-Semitism in America; Gil Geiss, a criminologist who gently critiqued my writing; Professor M., married to an undertaker's daughter, taught that there were two social strata, the living and the dead; Professor T., who kept a loaded pistol in our shared desk; Professor L., who moved to Detroit because his light-skinned children were becoming racists, somehow thinking that they were not black, too; and Professor H., who had joined AA and was "living one day at a time." I was the only woman in the department but, everyone else in the department, I felt, was the only one of their kind too. I never felt dissed, left out, or odd.

Teaching next at Denison University, I experienced college-wide colleagueship. I looked forward to our interdepartmental lunches. Faculty talked to each other and cared about each other. Students were bright and eager to change the world. And then there were the first years I taught at The Ohio State University, where the Women's Liberation movement brought lively graduate students to my department, and my cohort developed close friendships. I collaborated with two of them—Wen Li, from Taiwan, and Clyde Franklin, Jr., an African American from Memphis. Both of them have died, much too young.

Let me not get maudlin.

There are the continuing friendships I have with some of the women in my post-modernist-studies (PMS) group and with my co-conferees, and my actual and virtual graduate students. How fortunate I am.

I feel I should just stop here—stop on a positive note, but I can't. Too much stuff pounds in my head and heart.

Before I retired, the competition in my department for scarce rewards (salary increases, graduate students, teaching load, committee assignments, office space) had created an environment of envy, favoritism, and distrust. My department chair divided the faculty into three categories: outstanding, average, and poor. The outstanding received raises; average did not; and the poor paid more by having their teaching loads increased thereby insuring they would never pull themselves up by their mortarboard tassels. The faculty lounge, no longer "needed," was converted into a statistics-lab; a retirement party for a distinguished colleague was cancelled because no one was coming; and a trio of colleagues accused an outspoken Republican colleague of sexism and racism and had him brought before the university-wide Academic Misconduct Tribunal. Our dean kept a hit-list in her desk drawer—a list of faculty she would not support in any of their endeavors. He was on the list. I was, too. I think the Dean gave herself a bonus when I took the early retirement buy-out.

"Will we still be friends after I've retired?" I asked one of my closest academic buddies, a woman with whom I had shared two decades of theory-building and dinner conversations.

"Depends," she said. "On how organic it would be."

"Organic?"

"You know—still part of my work interest."

I asked another close academic friend the same question.

"Can't promise that, Laurel," she said. "Depends."

A decade has passed since those experiences and conversations, yet they still resound in my body.

The university I left has only gotten worse. The stereotype of the business world—step on the heads of others on your way to kissing the butt of the one ahead of you—is endemic. University problems are given to faculty committees, releasing the administrators with the bloated salaries from grunt work. Faculty morale plummets.

Students are "customers." Large class sizes mean more revenue. Faculty fear that the "customer is always right." One untenured faculty member who taught an on-line class was terrified that a student would lodge a complaint against her because she let four hours pass without answering an email. Such a complaint could jeopardize her hopes for tenure. In my last Sociology of Women's class, a trio of African American students walked out and reported me to the student tribunal because, as they said, I had no right to teach about blacks even though what I was teaching indicted whites. My own son Josh argues that because students pay for their classes, they have the right to show-up or not, come late or leave early, and to text during classes, or not.

Aren't I fortunate to be retired! I never thought I'd feel that with such conviction...

As I put to rest old wounds, I feel my spirits lifting.

I want to stay in this Family Room a while.

"Did I tell you about my friend Molly?" I am eavesdropping on a conversation between two fiftyish women, sisters-in-law perhaps, judging by the level of intimacy and distance. I love the story I overhear and can hardly wait to tell it to Ernest when he returns.

"I got you a box of fudge-centered ice-cream drumsticks," he announces. Getting the fudge-centered ones is a feat. We each start on one and I tell him about all that had gone on in this little enclave while he was out shopping.

"I'm so glad I'm out of the university," he says. Ernest retired twenty years ago at age fifty-two, after thirty years in academic life. When he finished grading his last class, he looked like a cat that had devoured an entire rookery. He said he felt like he had been released from prison. If he had to go back, now, I think he'd feel he was on death row. Twenty years later, and he is still smarting.

"Do you want to hear a story I overheard?" I ask.

"Talk-away."

"Well, this woman was talking about her friend Molly, an attorney married to an attorney. Molly home-schooled their two sons, both of whom wanted to grow up and become firemen. The older one did and the younger was set to follow in his brother's path. 'Jake, why not take the S.A.T.?' Molly asked nicely. Jake did. Scored at the ninety-ninth percentile. 'Why not apply to some colleges?' Molly asked even more nicely. He did and was accepted to them all. One university offered him a chance for a full four-year ride if he would come with his parents and be interviewed with twenty others in the auditorium with all the faculty and parents present. Only three would be offered the free ride. Chloe, the first candidate introduces herself and says she was valedictorian, went to Thailand with her church to help tsunami victims, won the free-style woman's championship in her state, and rescues greyhounds. The second candidate, Aaron, says he was the valedictorian of his eight hundred-member graduating class, won the state's science fair four times, composes and performs classical music on his cello, lute, violin and viola, raised $14,000 for Cat Welfare, and is an All-American sprinter."

"I get the picture," Ernest chuckles.

"So, it is Molly's son's turn. He says, 'Hi, I'm Jake . . . (long pause) . . . I taught myself how to juggle . . . Isn't this a clown college?' "

"*Run* by clowns!" Ernest says.

"Aren't they all?" I concur.

"So, I bet Jake got one of the scholarships," he says, chewing up the last of his drumstick.

"Yes. And I would have voted for him, too."

We walk the dogs back to my room, me on my walker holding Lily's leash. She doesn't pull. Ernest asks the nurse to put our two leftover drumsticks in the freezer. I am ready for a dog-nap.

Ring-ring.

"Hi Laurel . . . Patti, here." Patti is one of my academic friends from my feminist theory reading group. She comes from a South Dakota athletic family, and is large-boned, exuberant, and tough. She is a voracious reader of arcane postmodernist texts and a lightning rod for graduate students who want to be challenged. Some would call her charismatic.

"Hi, Patti."

"What say I come see you?…Bring you some….Thai?" About eighteen months ago, in the middle of a seminar she was teaching, she suffered a major hemorrhagic stroke on her left side. Two students caught her before she fell; another called 911; a third ran into another classroom to find an EMR certified person who came immediately to Patti's aid; and another had the emergency admissions at University hospital alerted. Patti spent five weeks in the hospital and another ten weeks in rehab at the University. I visited her several times in the hospital, but not in rehab, as I was warned that she had had an ICU psychosis, a not uncommon reaction to a lengthy stay in a rehab room without windows. The last time I saw her—about five months ago—it was painful to see her struggle with language, the blank look in her eyes, and the lack of animation in her face. She was affectless and scored so poorly on her executive functions evaluation that the doctor would not sign a release for her to drive. My intellectual colleague for thirty years was diagnosed with major cognitive problems.

"How 'bout night after next? Say at 5:00?" she asks. "I get tired early."

"Me, too." I say.

"What say I read you something I wrote? See if I'm getting better."

"Hi, Laurel," Jamal has come in. It is 8:30 p.m.

"Hi, Jamal."

"I'm sorry I have to weigh you again."

"Come back in half an hour, Jamal. I'm watching 'Dance Moms.'" Has it come to this?

"Hi, Laurel," Jamal has come back. It is 9:45.

"Can you come back in fifteen minutes? Now, I'm watching 'Project Runway.'" And this?

"Hi, Laurel." Jamal is back. It is 10:30.

I use my walker to get to the weigh station.

"Hmm. You've lost more weight," Jamal says.

We saunter back to my room, where Jamal two-steps around my table, picking up books, rifling their pages, putting them back down. He holds onto *Fearless Jones.*

"You can borrow that Walter Mosley book, if you want."

"Thanks, I've read it." Jamal looks sheepish

"Want to talk about it?"

"Well, I think, using the mystery genre featuring a Black book-dealer in Los Angeles in the 1950's tells me a lot about the Black experience back then . . . and tells me how a literary genre can teach history."

I don't tell him that my Uncle Morris was a book-dealer in Los Angeles in the 1950s, a friend of Mosley's, and a crusader who hired Black ex-convicts to convert them to communism.

"Oh, Jamal," I say, instead, "you are a good reader." To myself I say, Oh pul-eeze, Jamal, whatever you decide upon for your career, let it not be one in academia!

Food Good for Women

January 26

"You're not eating very much, are you Laurel?" Brooke has floated in with my breakfast tray. Has she read my chart?

"Just not very hungry," I say. "Dinner. Ugh—that's the worst."

"I think the food is better in the dining room. It's the same food, but the residents say it tastes better, fresher, because it is not on the steam trays. You might enjoy making friends with some of the residents here, too. You spend a lot of time in your room."

Brooke and I are at cross-currents. About the last thing I feel I need to do is make friends with any more residents. More and more, I love my time alone, looking out the window, thinking and being— things I don't seem to do when I am at home—always up and doing. But Brooke looks so ardent in her request. Maybe she knows something I don't know. Maybe she's concerned about my weight loss. Ernest and the dogs aren't coming tonight so I say, "Okay, I'll come to the dining room."

"Good. I'll tell the nurse." Brooke's voice swells with success. "The nurse will tell the dining room that you're coming. Come in at five and sit wherever you want." She straightens my plush coverlet and massages her engagement ring.

"So, getting married pretty soon? I ask.

"On Saturday! It'll be my day off."

"And your mom is well enough to come?"

"Um-hmm. It'll be a small wedding. That's what we want. Mom's making the cake."

"Hi, Trevor."

"Oh, Hi."

"I'll help you onto the NuStep," Prem, the East Indian physical therapist, says. I put both feet on the pedals and Prem adjusts the load to "2." "Push with both feet for two minutes," he orders, "and then three minutes with your good foot."

"Where's Colleen?" I ask.

"She's at school. She's taking a test today." Prem leaves me and goes to his desk. Exactly five minutes later he is back, smelling of sesame seeds. He asks, "Do you have stairs at home?"

"Yes."

"How many?"

"Isn't that information in my chart?"

"You need to reconfirm it," he directs.

I reconfirm that I have three concrete steps getting into my house, a flight of narrow steps to the shower, and another flight of steep stairs to the basement laundry room. I wish he would smile. "Is your family back yet?" I ask.

"Not yet." His black eyes widen, in surprise, I think, that I have re-membered. And then his face seems to darken again as he helps trans-fer me to my walker and walks with me to the free-standing staircase. "Today," he commands, "you'll walk up and down three steps."

"Follow me into the kitchen area," Melissa, the substitute occupa-tional therapist tells me.

"Where's Effie Lou?" I ask.

"She's taking a personal day."

I miss my regulars! How quickly I have become attached. *Desire the familiar.*

Melissa leads me on my walker into the therapy's "practice kitch-en." It has cupboards stocked with instant-foods, a sink with running water, a refrigerator and a microwave. It reminds me of the play kitchen I had when I was still a pre-schooler. Father had converted one of the basement storage rooms to hold my wooden kitchen appliances and my deep-blue painted table and chairs. There, I would hold tea parties with my dolls and my Rat Terrier, Happy. Father brought her home in a cardboard box on Christmas Eve when I was three and a half. I never thought of her as the family's dog. She was *mine*. I named her Happy after the dog in the Elson Readers. She slept with me and wore my hand-me-down dresses. The thought of Happy dying could always bring me to tears.

When I was a freshman in college, my mother phoned to tell me that Happy had been "put to sleep." Mother also told me that they had sold our Chicago house on Hermitage Avenue, bought a log-cabin house on Wonder Lake, and were moving to a three-room apartment on Sheridan Road. My Nancy Ann Story Book Dolls, children's books and various ephemera had been given to a "deserving little girl." After all this news, I sat, smoking, in the dorm's lounge, unable to cry. I was in shock.

"Are you paying attention?" Melissa demands. "I am going to show you how to make oatmeal."

"Oatmeal makes me throw up," I say. "I won't eat it."

"What about tea? Can you drink tea?" Melissa's holding her exasperation in check.

"I like tea."

She demonstrates how to take a tea-bag out of the box, and the bag out of its wrapper, and how to spoon in sugar and how to put the beverage into the microwave and how to turn the microwave on. "It's important," she opines, "to make sure the cup does not get too hot or you will burn yourself… Have you ever burnt yourself on a cup?"

Are we playing house here?

"Are you ready to try?" Melissa asks. Sugar would melt in her mouth.

"It's the refrigerator at home I'm concerned about," I say. "I'm not sure I can open it while I'm on my walker."

"Learning to use the microwave is first… refrigerator is later… we learn to master the kitchen in baby-steps."

I make the damn tea, hold it precariously as I baby-step myself to the table. I take a sip and gag.

"Hi Renee," I say. She is in her wheelchair heading toward the Therapy Room.

"Getting my prosthesis today," she chirps.

"Hi, Trevor."

Jingle-jangle.

Ernest puts Lily on Trevor's lap.

"Dog," he says.

Ernest takes Lily off Trevor's lap.

"Bye, dog," Trevor says.

"Hello. Hello. Hello. Hello." Beth from the Bingo game. She has a Hershey bar in her hand. "I have a camera…camera…dog picture…" She points the candy-bar at Bashi. He moves away. She pets Lily's back. Lily stands still. "Bye. Bye. Bye. Bye."

"Is that Lily?" Edna is in the hallway. "Lordy-mine, doesn't she look spiffy!"

"Read to me, Ernest," I ask.

"Food Good for Women?" he offers.

We laugh at this shared memory. Ernest is teaching-averse, and would have nightmares before the start of an academic year. One year he dreamed that he had been assigned a class entitled "Food Good for Women." He didn't know where the class was to meet and didn't have a syllabus. The only book he could think of was *Looking for Mr. Goodbar,* a novel about a woman who picks up men in bars. After sex, she tells her latest pick-up to leave because she's through with him. Of course, he murders her.

Ernest takes Lily and Bashi to the staff's break room to get himself a Diet Coke. Brooke had alerted us to the fact that their bottled drinks were half-the price of the ones in the Family Room. The staff will play with the dogs and then Ernest will take them out to the courtyard, where the smokers will blow smoke away from them, I hope. A little quiet time for me.

"Hey, Laurel." A voice from my past that I recognize but cannot identify.

"It's me—Ruth—from SalonLoft."

"Hi!" About five years ago, she completed her bachelor's degree and stopped cutting hair. Now, her hair is spiked, white and black, and buzzed up the back. I am excited to see her.

"I'm here to visit my aunt in the nursing home section, but I saw your name on the door as I passed by," she says. "What's going on?"

I tell her my tale. She tells me hers. Her aunt had moved to assisted living where she became increasingly unmotivated, demanding, and violent. On one evening visit, Ruth found her in a filthy bed, naked except for her soiled Depends. She was choking and gagging. Her temperature was 102. The squad took her to the hospital where surgeons penetrated her lungs and cleared out food debris, hoping they got all of it because its presence put her at risk for bacterial infection and pneumonia. She's still acting violently—throwing things at the nurses—but medically she's well enough to have been moved to a nursing home.

"I'm worried that she'll die here," Ruth says. "She's mean to the girls here. They'll either hurt her or ignore her."

I think of Vena and how she might hurt a violent and demanding resident, as she did Renee, or ignore one, as she did me my third night here, when phantom smells and touches put me into an angry panic.

"I wish there were a better option," I say, "for both resident and aide."

"Can I come in?" Renee is peeling a banana and crying at the same time. I bet she was one hell of a multi-tasker when she worked for the Feds.

"What's up?" I ask.

"My prosthesis."

"You got it?"

"I stood on it and it hurt too much. And that Rhonda was trying to make me stand back and that new one—Melissa—was helping her. Both of them pushing me around—just don't push me, don't push me, I told them—don't push my back—don't get behind me. I want to see you, see what you're doing—but they don't listen—they just treat me like a piece of rotten meat."

"I won't let Rhonda near me," I say.

"She's the worst."

"But could you stand on your prosthesis at all?"

"Three-seconds." Renee sniffs.

"Three-seconds! Why that's wonderful!" I say. "And the next time maybe it'll be seven seconds."

Jingle-jangle.

"C'mon Lily," Renee says. "Give me a kiss."

Five o'clock and I can hear the clattering of trays in the hallway. Time for me to head to the dining room. I wend my way past the tray-carts and the nursing station and turn right toward the dining room. At a table for four near the door sits Violet with six or so strands of popbeads around her neck; a blank-looking African-American man in a sports coat sits opposite her. Her husband? Her date? These two are the only African American residents I have seen. When I walk my walker towards them and nod to Violet, she bristles. She signals her displeasure with a palm down gesture, just like the "stay" gesture I use with my dogs.

"Join us. Join us. Join us." Bingo Beth is using the dogs' "come" gesture. Two other women are at her table, which is smack in the middle of the dining room. They each have plates, silverware, and water in their tumblers. The fourth place is not set.

"Hi, Beth," I say, sitting on the empty chair seat. "Hi, everyone. I'm Laurel."

"Mumble-mumble," says the white-haired woman across from me.

"You are-the-dog-lady," says the gray-haired woman next to me. I wonder if her medications flatten her voice.

"Lydia Lydia Lydia sits here here here," Beth tells me. "But she is sick sick sick."

"Here's your meds, Beth." A nurse watches as Beth swallows her pills.

"Who are you?" A young African American woman in a green uniform snaps at me. "What are you doing here?"

"I'm Room 112," I say, raising myself up on my haunches. "I asked to eat in the dining room tonight."

"You can't leave your walker like that," she says and abruptly walks away. A few minutes later she returns. "We've already sent your tray out."

"I want to eat here." My hackles are rising.

"Wait," she says, using the "wait" gesture I use with my dogs.

I wait. I had thought that the nurses' aides were the worst-off employees, now I wonder about the dining room staff. How little are they paid? How poorly are they treated by residents and supervisors? And no tips.

"Have some bread," Beth says. I think her meds have kicked in. "There are four slices and four butters," she informs me. "One, two, three, four."

"You can choose *mumble-mumble*," says white-haired woman.

"Not—all—the—time—," corrects gray-haired.

"This time only!" The wait-person sets my table place and pours my water.

"You can *mumble mumble*."

"Here—it—comes—late," announces gray-haired.

The wait-person wheels in our plates. Beth, gray-haired and I have fried chicken. White-haired has a gruel, and an elf-sized assistant in green who wields a mighty spoon.

"Bring your Paps to my room for a picture," Beth says. "Room 3947. I have a camera. I have a camera on my phone. Promise… promise… promise."

"Okay," I say. "I will."

"I do-not-like-dogs," gray-haired says.

"Not to worry," I say. "I won't bring them to your room."

"Mumble-mumble."

I look around the dining room. The minions of green elves and the lack of human conversations are eerie. I do not want this to be my future.

"We get coffee decaf coffee decaf," Beth tells me at the end of the meal.

"It—tastes—bad," gray-haired says.

"Mumble, mumble."

"No, you can't have any," the green elf says to the white-haired woman.

"I'll pass, too," I say. I get on my walker, leave my new-found "friends" and gratefully return to the privacy and cheer of my own room.

January 27

"How was your dinner in the dining room?" Brooke asks. She glimmers today like a koi in the sunlight.

"The food was better," I say. "But I prefer my own company."
Knock-knock.

"You have a special delivery package," says a chipper volunteer, old enough to be my mother. She brings it to my bed.

I open it. Ellyn has sent me Halvah! Comfort food! Chocolate sesame seed candy with pistachios! My mother used to buy it in half-pound slabs from the deli in Grandma's Russian Jewish neighborhood. We'd ride the El back home, sit at our green porcelain table and slather the halvah on Jewish rye-bread. Something I would eat, picky eater that I was. Still am. Slabs of fresh halvah are hard to come by here in central Ohio. I had told Ellyn I was lusting after it. She lives in Princeton; to get the halvah, she took the train to The Big Apple. (Why is New York City called that?) Or, maybe she had the sense to order by phone. Why haven't I thought of that?

Renee's door is closed.

"I'm glad you're back, Effie Lou."

Effie Lou sits me down, hands me three-pound weights for my hands, and puts two pound weights around my ankles. I sit-march and do bicep curls.

"That l'il Yorkie on-line I was tellin' ya'll 'bout." Effie Lou makes a sad face. "It's already bin boughten."

"Well, that's a bummer."

"But ah saw a l'il Pompoo at PetCorp. $400. I have in mind to jes git him. My step-son A. J. saw him. He sez he'll take a care of 'im if I hire him to. I think a l'il job'd be good for hiz self-esteem."

"I'm glad you're back, Colleen. How'd your test go?"

"I got a 'B'!" Colleen's beaming. "Competing against the younger ones, I did fine. I can move forward."

"What do you have in mind?"

"I'm thinking of becoming a surgical nurse. A lot easier than being a p.t."

"Easier?"

"Physically easier." Colleen shakes out her shoulders. "And emotionally easier, too. No one's sucking up to you or trying to suck out your energy. You don't have to order patients around, they're out cold. Okay, let's get you warmed-up on the NuStep... You'll have to come off, now, Violet. Laurel's scheduled... Remember, Violet, you should come late in the afternoon or very early in the morning."

Violet stares crossly at me. She's without popbeads this morning.

"I'm sorry," I say, putting my head down." It's not *my* fault, I am thinking, that the NuStep is reserved for the rehab patients, like the front seats of the Montgomery, Alabama busses were. Maybe, Violet, when you were riding in the rear, I was sitting-in at Chicago's Hyde Park Walgreens lunch counter, integrating it, or catching landlords in racist renting practices or maybe, a few years later, writing minutes and newspaper releases, and marching the streets of Los Angeles for the Congress of

Racial Equality. You don't know who I am, anymore than I know who you are. Are we not individuals to each other? Are we racial categories? "I'm sorry," I repeat. Sorry that you are so angry. Sorry that you have to be here the rest of your life. Sorry I don't know you. Sorry, sorry, sorry.

"I don't want to do the NuStep today," I say to Colleen. "I'm already warmed up. I just want to practice my stair-climbing."

"Okay, Violet." Colleen nods. "You can keep up your good NuStep work."

With Colleen at my side, I walk up and down four stairs four times on seventy-five percent weight. Down with the bad, up with good.

Renee's door is still closed. I hope she is okay.

Knock-knock.

"Come in."

Patti comes in with Thai carry-out and her bookbag. She is weak on her left side; her gait is awkward and her balance unsure. Just like me, I am thinking, but I will get better. Patti may never get better. For now, she has designed her own physical and occupation therapy.

"I am retrieving my mind," Patti says. "But, I'll never be one hundred percent."

"After my car accident and coma," I interject. "The neurologist said I lost about 10% of my smarts." I'm sure Patti has heard this story before, but she may not remember and it may be supportive because I know she thinks I'm still smart. Being smart, I think, has been the most important value in Patti's life. "But you know, Patti," I say, "that loss gave me greater access to my poetry-writing side."

"That's what people say, 'You close one door, it opens another.' "

I have never heard Patti utter a cliché. Maybe embracing "normal" talk will be her way back to "normalcy."

"So, how're you feeling now?" I ask.

"Grateful," she says.

I am surprised and happy to hear this. Is Patti uncovering parts of herself that have been buried under the weight of academia?

"Grateful," Patti repeats. "Grateful that I have come out of this so well. And, you know, Laurel, I'm still coming out of it. The idea that you have a year to recover is a bunch of shit. I still have surges of 'betterment.' "

We finish our Thai curries, and I return to my bed, set-up in sitting position. Patti sits in Ernest's comfy chair by the window. Lots of my visitors seem to prefer that chair. Is it the chair, the window, or the chair's placement? I think that not seeing the other's face head-on allows one to depend less on the other's response, letting one just say what they want to say.

I loved this about being in the car with my kids when they were riding in the passenger's seat. They'd talk and I'd listen. One of the most important conversations I ever had with Josh occurred in the car. He was seven years old and refused to go to school, saying he was sick. Because I didn't believe him, I drove him to the pediatrician, who declared that Josh was indeed sick with "Fifth's Disease"—a kid's kind of mononucleosis. "I wish you'd be like other moms," Josh said on our way home. My guilt about being a professor, instead of a stay-at-home mom like all the other mothers we knew was palpable. I'd been expecting this complaint for years. There was no research yet on how a mother's happiness affects her children, only psycho-analytical bromides blaming mothers for everything. "What do you mean?" I asked with trepidation. Josh looked straight-ahead and whispered, "Please, believe me when I tell you I'm sick." I breathed a sigh of relief, and said, "I will, if you promise not to pretend to be sick when you are not." I think the interaction in the car that day set up the possibility of trust between us, the possibility, ten years later, for me to trust Josh when he was on home-visit from his addiction treatment and for Josh to trust that I would trust him.

"Are you with me, Laurel?" Patti asks.

"Yep," I say.

"What say I read you my autobiographical sketch?" Patti takes a folder from her bookbag. "I think my brain's coming back."

"I love being read to," I say. I prepare myself for a disjointed or incomprehensible postmodernist essay. But what she reads is not only comprehensible and jargon-free, it is emotionally present and complex. In the first paragraph, she writes about her having an abortion and its relationship to her later feminist scholarship.

"It's wonderful, Patti." I've never known her to write about her personal life.

"I've been working on another piece, too," she says. "About athletes, but I'm not sure if I will be able to write it or publish it. "

"Too close to home?" I ask.

"Do we hire teachers or coaches?" asks Patti.

"Writing about the family has emotional risks," I say. "I'm still reeling from Cousin Barbara's assault regarding a paper I wrote twenty-five years ago. An assault on me and my father."

Patti and I discuss lies, erotics, families, and the locker-room in football, gymnastics, tennis, and synchronized swim. I give her my copy of Ernest's book, *Skeleton Key to the Suicide of My Father, Ross Lockridge, Jr.* "In that book," I tell her, "Ernest writes about the covert culture of child sexual abuse. How it is cocooned and protected and how it wreaks havoc."

Patti looks tired. "Do you think I'm recovering more from my stroke?" she asks.

"Indeed, you are." Patti and I have a history of being honest with each other. She can believe me.

Patti puts Ernest's book in her bookbag and takes out a linen-colored one. "Rosalind Krauss's book has helped me the most about my stroke," she says, handing me *Under Blue Cup.* I rub my fingers over its rough linen covers and smooth inserted drawing of a blue-trimmed cup atop a blue-trimmed saucer, both crazed. This is what a book should feel like, I think, the melding of tactile contradictions foreshadowing story. I cannot resist opening it: The first line hooks me: "Late in 1999, my brain erupted." I keep reading. The flow of blood from an aneurysm disconnected synopses and washed away neurons. Rosalind's short-term memory was compromised. She required cognitive training, like an athlete. One of the training exercises involved being shown unrelated pairs of objects—later words—and then twenty minutes later to tell the evaluator what the objects were. The first success that Rosalind had with words was "under blue cup." She could succeed because they reverberated with her *long term* memory; she could link the disparate words into one meaningful sentence from her past. Remembering *who she was* and *what she had experienced in her early life* gave her a route into settling into and rebuilding her current life. "Thus," she writes, "the aneurysm thrust forgetting into my experience as a possibility I'd never imagined."

"You can keep the book here, if you want," Patti says as she gathers her stuff together and walks toward the door.

I am tired, too, but grateful that, like Patti, I never experienced any childhood sexual abuse. I begin to ruminate on that and the scary feeling that catches me now and then, catches me now. All the talk about memory, knowing who you are and what you experienced is chomping at my body. The bits of memory; the experience I have never talked about to anyone. The lingering feeling of being "bad." I was just a little girl, maybe three or four, wearing a pinafore. My father was with some men on the porch of the farmhouse when I wandered off into the cornfield. I got lost and began to cry. It seemed as if I would never be found, when a man finally did find me. He put his hand under the top of my pinafore, squeezing my little nipples. He said something like I shouldn't "show" myself—and some other stuff I can't remember.

Ring-ring.
"Hi, Honey." It's Barrie. "Is this a good time?"
"The best," I say. We chat a bit, and then I ask, "Do you remember me being lost at a farm?" The scariness is all around me.
"Yeah. We'd gone for corn." Barrie says.
"Do you remember who found me?"
"Let me think…yeah…Uncle Pete."
"Cousin Barbara's father?"
"Yeah. Why are you thinking of that?"

I am not *retrieving* the memory. I never lost it. I just didn't know who the perpetrator was. Now that I do, I can begin to make some sense of that which has not made sense. My entire childhood I was on guard around Uncle Pete, never willing to be alone with him. Mother never made me sit next to him at the table or on the couch, or, for that matter, talk to him. Most of my life, I have doubted whether he really was my father's brother. The story we were told was that when they were children my father and his sisters went to live with Great Aunt Ruby. "Baby Pete" went to live with the Draco family, a family we never met. When Father was in the cavalry in Texas, a Gypsy fortune-teller told him to go to the Addison Avenue Tavern in Chicago where he would meet his little brother, Pete, a brother he didn't know he had. Pete wheedled his way into my parents' life. I am willing to believe miraculous stories told by psychics, but I never bought this story. *Why?* Because I do not want Pete to be my uncle.

I can build such a case against him, and to do so feels both childish and redemptive.

On holidays, my family would first spend time with Pete's family, and then spend time with our other relatives. Pete's family was never included. I knew there had been some rift, but now I think it probably had to with Pete acting inappropriately towards my girl cousins. Did he molest his own daughters, too? I think that is why they all shared a bedroom, one of them sleeping in a baby-crib with the sides up, until she got married.

I think, now as I write this, that there is no such thing as a "little" molestation. Beginning with my pre-school years and up to the present, the cornfield event has impacted my life. When I was still a pre-schooler, I would choose not to swim rather than go topless. I never again wore pinafores or any garment where my chest could be seen from above or sideways. In grade school, I learned how to take off my shirt and put on my bathing suit or pajama top without exposing my chest, lest, God,—that "dirty old man"—see me. In middle- school, my fear was palpable whenever a boy flicked the back of my bra—*ha-ha!* I sharp-elbowed one zealous boy in the stomach for which I was remanded to Principal Flynn's office. Too embarrassed to tell her what had provoked my assault, I was required to write, "I am sorry for my bad behavior" five hundred times. In high school, I wore hard-feeling falsies, not so much to increase my size as to have a barrier between me and the wandering hands of my dates. As an adult, I have never shown cleavage or accented breast shape. Here in the Bellemont, my breast shyness manifests in my avoidance of being bathed by the staff.

My reading has been affected, too. I don't read about childhood trauma, in general, or rape or sexual abuse, in particular. I do not even like writing those words. Or reading them . . . when I tried to read William Faulkner's' novel, *Sanctuary,* I could not get past the girl's rape with a corncob. In my mind, that fictional rape occurred in the cornfield—

I *need* to write my cousin Barbara:

Dear Barbara,

Recovering from my ankle surgery is going to be a slow and painful process. The doctor says at least a year—maybe eighteen months. I need to build my strength and preserve my energy.

I am not up to listening to your pain and anger about my sociological work published a quarter century ago. I wrote what I thought was the truth. I would never purposely hurt you.

I remember what your father did to me and that he must have done similar things to other girls. This explains a lot about my life that I did not understand until now.

Your lashing out at my father is unacceptable.

So, I think any phone-call is yours to make. When you feel you want to just chat with me—then I welcome hearing your voice, and hearing how your house-hunting, life, and times, are going.

Love,
Laurel

Jingle-jangle.

"Yap-yap-yap."

"Oh, Ernest. Thanks for coming tonight. I need a kiss."
"Yap-yap-yap."
"Oh, Pappidinkers! I love you so!!"
"Ernest, will you mail this letter to Barbara for me?"

My breathing feels more open, chest most expanded.

CHAPTER 12

Training Wheels

January 28

Renee's door is open and I walk my walker in. "Good Morning, Renee. Your door was closed all day yesterday. Are you okay?"

"I don't think I'm going to make it, Laurel." She pulls her head back into her shell. Her long dark hair fans out around her face. "The prosthesis hurts too much."

I want to tell her about Tami's father's double-amputations, and how he decided to forego his prostheses, preferring his wheelchair— and how he made a new life for himself in the nursing home, getting re-married to a fellow resident, enjoying his life. But I don't. Someone else's success is irrelevant. Instead I say, "I'm so sorry for your pain, Renee, but I do think you will make it."

"You do?" Renee brightens up.

"You are a survivor."

"I am that. A survivor."

"Hi, Trevor."

"Dogs…dogs…dogs."

"Later, Trevor."

"C'mon, Laurel 'n take a lookie-see at my Pompoo." Effie Lou is holding her iPhone and calling me over to her desk. "We git her last night and named her 'Shelby' after my county in Kin-tuc-ky."

"What a darling little dog," I say. I don't comment on the name. My poor Lily had belonged to at least three different breeder/owners before she got her forever home with us. Shelby was Lily's name when we got her, and before that it was Miranda. She shuddered when we said "Shelby," and lowered her tail when we said "Miranda." We'll never do that "name-calling" again.

"Shelby's goin' sleep with me. Tony is on a toot. His ma dunno whaz-up either."

"Big day for you today," Colleen says. She stretches out her back. "Take a seat, you're going to get your training wheels!" Colleen turns my walker over, goes into the supply closet and comes out empty-handed. "Anyone see the wheels for Laurel's walker?"

"Sure haven't," says Rhonda. She's raising her shoulders up to her ears. She looks a little too gleeful. Others shake their heads.

"Looks like I'll have to borrow some from this other walker," Colleen says.

Foiled again, Rhonda!

Colleen bolts the cannibalized wheels to my walker. "Note, that the wheels are on the insides of the legs," she says. "Not the outsides where they catch on things and make the walker even wider. Not all therapists know *that*."

"How do you know so much?"

"Twenty-seven years of experience," Colleen says.

I knew she would say that and I wanted her to have the opportunity to brag.

Colleen explains how to use the wheeled walker, and I go on my first test-run up the hallway. This is so much easier than the "step and stop and pick-up walker" routine. Not as much fun as the scooter, but quite exhilarating. "Be sure to always keep your feet inside the walker's perimeter," Colleen instructs, noting my desire to wheel away, faster and faster. For some inexplicable reason, this change has not made me anxious. Maybe because I am familiar with the walker, itself, and because the wheel-controls are like the scooter's. How nice not to be a wimp.

"Hi, Edna," I say, passing her room. She's only been here a couple of days and already has a wheeled walker. Rehab from a hip replacement is so much faster. For that matter, so is knee replacement, heart surgery, childbirth, cataracts, and tonsillectomies.

"Hi, Dearie," Edna says. "Now don't get any speeding tickets, youngster."

"I'll try my best," I say.

Fifty years ago, California's driving law stated that one drove the posted speed limit *or* a speed "appropriate for the driving conditions." I was driving my Morris Minor with red-racing stripes at its top speedometer speed of 72 mph, trying to keep up with the traffic that was crowding me on the freeway. A police officer picked me out and ticketed me because I was going over the 65 mph limit. He ticked me off. So, I went to court and argued given the "conditions" under which I was driving, it was "appropriate" for me to speed up to reduce the probability of a multi-car accident. The bar-certified lawyers in court laughed at me—a girl arguing her own case. I was twenty. I won. I did not have to pay an exorbitant ticket or court costs, and California rewrote its law. Now, no matter the conditions, you cannot drive *faster* than the posted speed. *Mea Culpa.*

Some twenty-years ago an apologetic Worthington police officer ticketed me for going 27 mph in a 25 mile zone ... my own neighborhood. "Sorry," he said. "I have to apply the law the same to everyone." I paid my fine in mayor's court, and my neighbors have ever since been saved from my recklessness .

Renee's in the hallway in her wheelchair, pumping her one partial leg.

"Good to see you up and about," I say and then cringe at my lack of language sensitivity.

"I've been thinking," Renee says. "I need a dog."

"A service dog would be great," I say.

Renee cocks her head. "You know how child protective services take children away from abusing parents?"

"Yes."

"I wonder if there is a dog protection agency to take abused dogs away—you know, how you might be reported for abusing Lily—and then, do you think the agency would give Lily to the person who reported the abuse?"

I can't tell if Renee is serious . . .

"Ready for your prosthesis therapy, Renee?" Rhonda has appeared.

"No!" Renee yells. "I don't feel well." She wheels herself back into her room and shuts her door.

Rhonda looks like *she* is about to cry. "I am really not cut out for this kind of work," she says to me.

"Not your favorite job," I say, surprised at Rhonda's candidness.

"I'm used to being good at what I do." She raises her shoulders. "I'm really good at weight-training elite athletes." Rhonda pretend jerks and lifts an imaginary barbell.

"Were you a competitive weightlifter?" I ask, noting her stance, explosive energy and grace.

"Won 'Best Lifter' in a dozen competitions."

"We rehabbers as clients—not so good, huh?"

"We're not the best team." Rhonda chortles. "And I'm not show-ing improvement, so I guess I'd better leave. Actually, I'll only be at the Bellemont for another two weeks. I've got a gym-backer. I'll be training athletes and being coached myself . . . who knows . . . maybe I'll be in the next Olympics."

"I bet you will," I say. "You're Rhonda-the-Strongest."

Jingle-jangle.

"Look at me!" I say, wheeling towards the Paps coming down the hallway.

"Dog dog dog," says Trevor.

"Well, just look at you!" Ernest says, admiring my wheels.

"Dog dog dog." Trevor says, pointing at Lily.

Ernest puts Lily on Trevor's lap. Trevor does not try to get up, but tentatively pats Lily on her head. That's her sweet spot.

Bashi starts yapping his head off and pulling on his leash. I see why. He sees another dog, an Irish Setter in a Delta Therapy Dog vest, leashed to a rigid woman wearing a Pendleton vest.

"Leave it, Bashi," I command. "No pulling…Leave it…Good quiet dog!"

The woman's body gets even more rigid, military. She looks forlorn.

"I want my dogs to be certified therapy dogs, too," I say, trying to start up a conversation. "Can you tell me about Delta?"

"This is only my second time at the Bellemont," she says as if that is somehow relevant. I wonder if I will look as forsaken as she does if I come with my dogs to a nursing home, not knowing anyone special, not having anything more personal to do. And if I became a Delta certified handler, would I have to take on that military bearing—the stance that the Dog-Whisperer says conveys that you are leader of the pack?

"Would you like your dog to meet my other dog?" I ask, pointing to Lily doing her amateur therapy work on Trevor's lap. "She's less hyper."

"Thank-you, No." The woman makes no eye-contact. "I'll just wait until someone asks for Skipper."

It is a sunny day, a kind of January thaw day, and I decide I would like to walk my wheeled walker outside into the courtyard where the dogs can romp and I can sit on a lawn chair in the fresh air, breathing in the second-hand smoke of the staff, visitors, and residents. I'll pretend I am at a barbeque. A mostly toothless, small and wrinkled man is here smoking Marlboros and wearing a tight-fitting deep purple T-shirt. It says:

I look like twenty.
I feel like sixty.
I act like thirty.
I must be forty.

I laugh. He looks ninety! Maybe he's only fifty? Two women are on oxygen, and smoking. Renee's daughter Miranda and grand-daughter Jody are here.

"Do you want to pet Bashi?" Ernest asks Jody.

"Apache," Jody says, petting Bashi's right flank. His sweet spot. "Does Apache have a visible fence?"

"He does," Ernest says.

Miranda offers me a Camel. I decline.

I learned to smoke in Anshe Emet Sunday School. Rather than going to class, I would smoke with the older girls in the bathroom. I was twelve. I furthered my addiction at Presbyterian Family Camp where I would smoke with the older kids on the back-side of a barn, out of sight of our parents. I was thirteen. In high school, when father threatened to send me to reformatory school, for reasons other than smoking, all I could think of was could I smoke there. Going to college at a young age let me increase my consumption. I had rules I followed, like not smoking before lunch. But that meant staying up late playing bridge and smoking. Another rule was not to inhale. *Who was I kidding*?

For a quarter of a century, I smoked when I was happy, sad, scared, tired, hungry, angry, relieved, full, thirsty, quenched, bored, anxious, depressed, alone, not alone. My addiction was so awful that I would do almost anything to get my fix, although I would never have called it that. I drove in snow-storms and thunderstorms to the carry-out, on occasion leaving my children at home alone. I asked strangers for lights. If there had been a party at my house and my good-hostess manners forced me into sharing my Benson & Hedges until none were left, I would re-light any butts of any brand I found in the ashtrays. Ernest and I would stick straight-pins in butts so we could get enough distance to get the last lick of tobacco out of it and into our stupid mouths.

About thirty-years ago, the Lung Association, in collaboration with the exercise-physiology program at Ohio State University, offered faculty a quit-smoking program. First, you had to pass a heart test. I did. Ernest did not. Then, you had to exercise rather than smoke. Most of the enrollees dropped out. Ernest and I had tried to quit separately, but that didn't work because we would take drags off the cigarettes of the one still smoking. So, Ernest did the program, unofficially. We put rubber-bands around our wrists and snapped them hard whenever we wanted a ciga-rette. We spent a lot of time in non-smoking places. We learned that the urge to smoke passed after a few minutes and that the urge came less and less frequently. We were the only ones doing the program who success-fully quit. My best friend Betty never quit. Emphysema killed her. My sister quit five months before she died of lung and colon cancers.

"Ernest, I am so glad that we quit smoking when we did."

"It's harder for folks, now," Ernest says. "So many addicting addi-tives."

"I wonder what's been added to cigarettes now."

"Chocolate, for one."

"Good idea," I say. "Time for a chocolate-fudge ice-cream drum-stick."

We return to the nurses' station, dogs in tow. We look in the refrig-erator for our drumsticks. They're gone! Vanished! Stolen?

"Maybe whoever took them is a chocolate addict," I say. "Or, just a thief."

"How much would you say a dog like Lily would cost?" Renee asks. She's in the hallway.

"There's a Papillon rescue group," I say. "You can find it on the Web."

"But it won't be Lily, will it?"

"Maybe sort of like her," I say.

"I'm going to have a big settlement. My lawyer's coming next week." Renee assesses me and then Ernest. "How much would you sell Lily for?"

"Sorry, she's not for sale," Ernest says.

"C'mon, how much?"

"Not for sale!" I say.

Renee wheels herself back into her room muttering. Slams the door.

January 29

This is my first trip on my wheeled walker to the beauty shop—and my last. Walking through the long-term and dementia wards brings me to tears. From the sights, sounds, and smells, I could be in Calcutta or Petrozavodsk, not just around the corner from where I bed down in rehab, and just a seven-minute drive from where I live. Or, I could be in an archaic insane asylum, "the snake pit"—where patients scream, "Help me... Help me...," spit and drool and *look* crazy with their blank stares, chewed finger nails, and uncombed hair, even if they aren't. A friend's husband is here. He asks her, "Am I going to be here until I die?" She answers, "No one knows when they're going to die." She prays that he "passes over" soon, though, and feels guilty about her prayers.

"No thanks," I say to the Bingo players. "Not today."
"Good good good prizes!" Bingo Beth says.

"Hi, Laurel." Mildred is ready for me.
"My last hair wash here." I settle into a distressed chair. "I'm going home this week."
"You can come back to me, if you want, after you're discharged," Mildred says.

I take my wheeled walker back through the long term ward. I hold my breath as best I can so as not to smell the smells. I look for Room 3937 so I'll know where to take the Papillons to have their pictures taken by Beth, but I can't find the room. I peek into Room 397, thinking that might be Beth's room. It isn't. There's an old woman on her back calling out, "Kiss me... Kiss me." *She isn't asking for much.* In the bed next to her an old man is sleeping. Probably her husband. I wonder how often spouses end up together in long-term wards. I air-blow her a kiss.

I wheel on and peek into Randy's sister's room, but she appears to be asleep. A quiz show is on her television. A soap opera is on her roommate's set. When I close my eyes, my ears open wider to the cacophony of phony television voices. I want to scream—I want to hear myself scream—I want these residents to hear a live woman's voice, unfiltered though boxes with wires. No, what I want is to move quickly through this ward and get to the Therapy Room.

"Hi, Colleen!" I am glad to see her looking less strained. Her back pain appears to be less burdensome.

"NuStep for you," Colleen says. "I think you're ready for 100 percent weight bearing."

"Am I?"

"Let's try you." Colleen adjusts the NuStep to "1" and I put both feet on their pedals. I feel uncertain.

"It's okay. Push down. You can do it, Laurel."

I push. Colleen sets the timer for three minutes.

"Get on your walker," Colleen instructs. "We're heading toward the basement."

"What?"

"Today you did so well on the NuStep that I'm advancing you to the basement stairs."

"No way."

"Yes, way."

Colleen walks with me out into the corridor, past the greeter's booth and we stand beside a wide door I had not noticed before. There is a yellow Caution sign on it. She opens it and I peer into a small metal landing and a set of wide metal steps leading into a dark basement space. Metal banisters protrude from the walls beside the steps—which seem to be getting steeper and slipperier the longer I look at them. My heart is pounding.

"What's down there?" I ask. When I was three, I got lost in the basement of a large apartment complex that had wire cages filled with boxes and spiderwebs. I screamed and cried and waited forever until I was found by a nice man and his wife. They lived in the basement.

He was our janitor. She gave me cookies and milk. Ever after—as long as we lived in that apartment building—I found my way back to their apartment. I felt safe there.

"We keep storage down there," Colleen says matter-of-factly.

"What's that noise?" I ask. "Sounds like a B-52 bomber taking off—or landing."

"That's our industrial washing machine."

"'Scuse us." Two nurses' aides come up the stairs and out the door.

"Hi," I say, although I do not recognize the women. Maybe they're new. They probably work in the unskilled sections, and maybe they've had a nice little break together in this basement. I hope so. I hope, too, that there aren't any spiders down there.

"Ready, Laurel?" Colleen has me walk my walker onto the metal landing and asks me to leave it there, hold onto her shoulder and hop over to the steps on my good foot. I grab the left banister. It feels as though time has slowed down while my heart rushes on. All I can see are the steep stairs in front of me. I am frozen. I doubt if I can get down them without tumbling arse over teakettle, as someone use to say. I don't remember who. I can't concentrate.

"You can do it," Colleen croons. "Remember 'down with the bad.' It's just like the stairs in the Therapy Room, only more of them. Put your bad foot down and then put your good foot on the same step. Hold onto the banister. I'll be in front of you... You won't fall."

Tentatively, I begin my descent. This descent is not, I convince myself, as challenging as the Grand Canyon's North Kaibab trail that Ernest and I attacked in mid-day, planning on finding fresh water at the river, only to find that the mules had used the water as a toilet; on the ascent, heat-stroke struck me—fortunately only a few yards from a spring, from which Ernest brought water and brought me back from semi-unconsciousness.

"You're doing great!" Colleen coaches me. "Keep coming... You're almost down... Great job!...Rest a bit, before you start up....I've brought you a water-bottle... Drink up... Rest."

"Okay," I say. "I'm ready to start up... up with the good..."

"There you are." Effie Lou is waiting in the corridor for me.

"I think she's done enough for the day," Colleen says. "She did good."

"I'll walk 'er back." Effie Lou looks worn-out.

"How's your puppy doing?" I ask as we start the trek back to my room.

"Shelby's jes scrumptious. She's flat-cold good 'bout doin' her biz-ness outside."

We get to my room. "It's Tony," she says, closing the door.

I'm expecting to hear he's abusing Effie Lou and Shelby.

"It's hiz ball. Swelled bigger than a base-ball. Hard like a base-ball. He's in cryin' out loud pain and won't let me near him."

"Oh, Effie Lou!"

"I tell him he's gotta see the doc. So, he's goin' today but he don't wan' me to go with him. He'll call. He sez he will."

Jingle-jangle.

"Yap. Yap. Yap."

I wheel myself into the corridor to greet my Paps.

"Hi, Trevor," Ernest says.

"Lil-lee . . . Lil-lee . . . Lil-lee."

"Here she is," Ernest says, putting Lily on Trevor's lap. I think it re-markable that Trevor has asked for her by name, but none of the nurses writing at their desks, seem to have noticed.

"I brought you some ice-cream drumsticks," Ernest says. He gives me one and puts the others in the nurses' refrigerator.

"See you later, Trevor," I say.

"Carry Lily?" Ernest says, taking Lily into his arms.

"Yap-Yap," Lily says.

"Yap-Yap," Bashi says, which I think means, *What about "carry me?"*

"Ready for your shower?" Nurses' aide Vena is at my door, softly humming a Christian spiritual. Sounds like *Are You Washed in the Blood*, but maybe not. Today Vena does not look angry.

"How are you?" I ask.

"It's all good," she says. "Got my car fixed…got my skilled-ward back…maybe I'll get a raise…got my kids talking to me…And how about you, Laurel?"

"I'm good," I say. "I'm not sure I want a shower, though."

"I'd like you to," Vena says. There is a pleading in her voice. Maybe her raise depends on my taking a shower?

"Have you used these before?" I ask, pointing to my DryPro Cast Cover.

Vena reads the directions and quickly puts my leg in its Drypro. "Clever," she says, as she pumps the air out. "Never saw one of these before." I am thinking that Vena is undervalued here, underemployed, undereducated and that there is not a damn thing I can do about it—other than be appreciative.

"Vena, you put that cast cover on better than the occupational therapist! Thanks."

"You're welcome." Vena and I are actually having a civil conversation. *How nice!*

I gather together life's blessings—no, that's what Vena is humming—I gather together my robe and clean clothes. She helps me into my wheelchair and wheels me to a Shower Room in the corner by the long-term wards.

"Do they have separate showers for men and women?" I ask. I don't think it's an idle question as I look around me at the desexualized bodies in shapeless clothing, slumped in their wheelchairs. Would "sex" be a last identity to be honored in a nursing home—even if the resident didn't know or care?

Vena uses her key to open the room. It's occupied, she says with a man, and 'yes' we keep the men and women separate. But, there's another shower room near the nurses' station. It's not as easy to use, but it'll work.

Vena pushes me back to the short-term rehab ward to an unlabelled door near the staff break room. She opens the door and pushes my chair into the auxiliary shower. The room, a dark high-ceilinged cement-floored and cinder-blocked open space, feels vast to me—large enough to simultaneously shower fifty or one-hundred inmates—like the "showers" at Auschwitz where Jewish people were gassed en masse. I learned about those showers when I was a six-year old in Sunday School at Anshe Emet, the same year I got showered at a public pool, feet irradiated in green goo, and, collapsed from heat-stroke. To this day, I don't like to shower in hotels and I refuse to see *Psycho.*

Vena helps me undress, politely averting her eyes from my aging body, protecting me from embarrassment. She helps me transfer to a plastic shower-chair with rows of holes in its seat. It is positioned under a hand-held shower and over a large drain-hole. If I were a little girl, I would worry I would fall down that hole, like I used to worry about the bath-tub drain, or I would remember when my brother put me down a sewer hole and stepped on my hands hoping I would fall in and be forever gone from his life, but my father saved me—but I am not a little girl, and wonder of wonders, I do not feel vulnerable either to the drain or the shower, which is now sprinkling my shoulders, torso, and legs in a perfect tepid temperature and spray. Sitting in my plastic shower-chair, I feel safe, caressed by the water and tended to by a Sierra Leone *angel.*

"Take as long as you like," Vena says. "There is no hurry." She leans back in a chair and hums, *"Down by the river."*

"Sing it, Vena! Sing it!"

How soothing! Me in a shower listening to a Vena concert. Me, not skittish or scared. By- and-by, my alto harmonizing with Vena's soprano. *"I'm goin' lay down my sword and shield."* Vena pats me dry and transfers me to my wheelchair. I get dressed and she leisurely wheels me back to my room.

A skinny white woman in a business suit is my room, sitting at my table, tapping her foot. She flashes her ID at me and hands me her card: Geri Sanderly—LifeHomeCare. She asks me to join her at my table, but I decline. I am tired from my shower. I stretch out on my bed.

"It will be harder for me to fill in the forms if you aren't at the table." Geri frowns. She cannot keep the annoyance out of her voice.

I shrug.

"For the first month you are home, you are entitled to three times a week visits from a home physical therapist and a home health aide." She is speaking rapidly. "The aide will help you with your personal needs."

"What's included in personal needs?" I ask.

"Bathing…laundry…putting clothes away…microwaving food…light house-keeping."

"Dog walking?"

"No!" She fills out her paper-work.

"Do you like your job?" I ask. She seems so unhappy.

Ignoring my question, Geri gets up and brings the paperwork to my bedside. "Sign here. . . and here…and…here." She packs it up. "The manager told me you'd be here when I came and you weren't. I am running late for my next appointment. I'll get written-up. Oh, and LifeHomeCare thanks you for choosing them."

January 30

Brooke glides in with my breakfast and straightens up my room. Her usually wayward tendrils are slicked back. Her face glows. Soon she will wed, but I do not think her life will alter greatly. She will still be a nurses' aide, still be in school, still have an ill mother, and still be glistening—I hope.

"How's everything going?" Brandon is at the door. He looks spiffy in his shades of brown co-ordinated clothing.

"You look spiffy," I say.

"Thanks. Kohl's had a good sale."

"Anybody helping out Renee?" I ask.

"We've had a meeting about her," Brandon says, and stops, being careful, I think, not to violate patient privacy.

"The woman in Room 3947 wanted to take pictures of my dogs, but I couldn't find the room," I say.

"We don't have a room with that number," Brandon says.

"She was so sure . . . I bet that's her home address number."

"Do you know her name? Maybe I can locate her."

"Hmm . . . Beth . . . ?"

I toss my blue-ski jacket into the basket of my walker and start up the corridor. My neighbor Edna's door is open, and I peek into her room. Fresh yellow irises on her Chantilly lace covered tablecloth. Antique silver framed photographs encircle the flowers. The bed sheets and pillows are pink and flowery. She's wearing a plush lavender outfit, sitting on a chair covered with a mauve throw, and reading a hard-covered book, whose title I cannot see. It looks like she has made herself at home.

"How're you doing, Edna?" I ask. "Your room looks so homey."

"Dearie-me," Edna says, "I am fine. My husband brought me new irises. Aren't they the nicest? I told him what linens to bring from home. I like the 900 count threads better than what we have here. So, he did bring them and Brooke—do you know Brooke, the nice aide?"

"Yes, I like Brooke."

"Well, Brooke remade my bed with my sheets from home. Isn't she a dear? And she set up the table décor—of course, I told her where to put things—you know she's young and has not been in charge of a house yet so I think I've helped her get on in her life."

"The lace cloth is lovely," I interject.

"That table! Lordie-lord! Have you ever seen a more scratched up piece of furniture in your life? You should have your hubby bring you a table-cloth for your table. Or, I can ask my husband to bring one for you. Would you like that, dearie?"

"Thanks," I say. "I'm fine. I'll be going home soon." I am not going to get chummy again with Edna.

"Hi, Trevor." He's in the corridor in his tailored pajamas in his wheelchair. He looks asleep. I like Trevor. Effie Lou meets me in the corridor. I ask, "Any news about Tony?"

"He's gettin' a biopsy this afternoon. He's scared."

"How're you doin?"

"Tony wants me to git pregnant now—jes in case—but Ah told him 'uh-uh.' My doc sez Ah need to lose seventy pounds before Ah get pregnant. I'm on a diet now and it'll take two years to do it right. Ahv 'ready lost five pounds."

"I've noticed," I say. "Good for you."

"Ahm bringin' Tony to the doc. Hiz mom will have to take off work and pick up A. J. from school and A. J. will have to let the puppies out case we are real late."

"Laurel, you wait in the sitting area." Colleen has met us in the corridor. "I'll get my SUV."

"Bye-now," Effie Lou says.

I give her a big hug.

"You going some vere?" Ilsa asks in her German accent. I remember the trouble she was having with her foot brace in the Therapy Room, but we have never talked. The brace looks tightly laced as she swings her foot. Her fur coat is open at the neck. She is on the couch in the sitting area.

"Colleen is going to teach me how to transfer from my walker into a car seat so I can go for a home evaluation tomorrow." This is probably more than Ilsa wants to know.

"They vant to evaluate my house, too," Ilsa says. "I don't vant them crawling all over my place looking into everything of mine."

"You don't have to have them come," I say. "It's voluntary. It's your choice." Ilsa brings out the contrariness in me. Her looks, accent and demeanor put me in mind of an SS concentration camp guard. The staff don't like her. I've heard them talk about her behind her back. I think she's probably racist.

"So, what happened to your foot?" I ask, trying to be friendly.

"*They* did it!" Ilsa stares at me. "Don't you know vat happened?"

"No."

Ilsa seems to be assessing my veracity.

I shrug my shoulders.

"I vas here visiting my friend who vas here recovering from a broken hip. I vas standing still ven I got hit with a laundry cart—being pushed backwards. It knocked me over and my femur and ankle vere broken. I am suing them."

"Terrible," I say.

"Yah."

"But you came back here for your therapy?" I try to modulate my incredulity.

"It is the best place for therapy." She raises her eyebrows and taps her thigh. "Don't you know that?"

"No, I didn't," I say. She must think I'm an idiot.

"But they have to like you." Ilsa squints at me. "I've seen you in the Therapy Room. They like you. But they don't like me."

I think Ilsa has that one right. She always seems discontented and angry. Staff avoid her.

"Staff avoid me," Ilsa says. "They know I can sue for other things, too . . . maybe sue one of them . . . so they don't vant to help me. But, now, if I don't let them evaluate my house, they say they vill be absented from any problems I might have in the future." Ilsa is spitting angry. "So, vat choice do I have? None. I have to let them into my house."

"Are you ready?" A tall, dark, and handsome African American man with a military bearing touches Ilsa on her shoulder.

"Meet my husband, Americus," Ilsa says. "He's taking me shopping."

Americus smiles. His teeth gleam.

"All set?" Colleen has come in. I put on my jacket, glad to have something to do to quiet my anxiety. I can see the cement under the awning. It looks slippery to me. Will my wheels hold? Will I fall? . . . *I do have brakes . . . And Colleen will be there . . .* I read somewhere that when adrenaline surges, the fight or flight response sets in. Whether you are a fighter or a flighter seems to mirror how you are when the adrenaline is not flowing. I am conflict and risk-adverse. I think I am a flighter by nature. In college, one of our favorite games was to imagine how it is we would go crazy. I always imagined myself in a catatonic state, sitting on a window-seat with my legs pulled up, chin on my knees, my eyes blank—

"Let's go!" Colleen is beside me and we walk out to her SUV. The cement is not slippery.

"We don't have SUV's," I say. "We have sedans."

"It's the same procedure. It's no different, actually, than transferring from the walker to your bed or wheelchair."

I hold onto the SUV"s passenger door, crouch down and sit. *Worrying about it was much worse than doing it.*

"Where's Trevor?" I ask the nurse behind the counter.

"He be getting his shower," she says, without looking at me.

"Going home soon to your pool?" I'm visiting in Renee's room. Her daughter Miranda is there.

"We don't have a pool!" I say.

"But you're rich," she says. "You're writers."

"Writers aren't rich, Ma," Miranda says.

"A couple of them—like Stephen King are—but we're *not* rich."

"You had a tiger-lined coat."

"I was a kid."

"You have those expensive dogs." Renee narrows her eyes.

"We got them on the cheap," I say, "because they weren't good enough to be champion show dogs in America." I am equivocating.

"Ma, I don't think they cost all that much."

I am glad that Miranda is here.

"Well, I've got to get some groceries on my way home." Miranda leans down and kisses her mother's head and waves good-bye to me.

"Your dad talked to me about your sister," I say to Renee.

"To *you*?"

"Yes…"

"Did he use my sister's name?"

"Yes."

"He never uses her name around me. He never talks about her to me. My mother took all the pictures of her down. She acts like Donna never lived."

"How sad."

"And now that's goin' to happen about me, too. I've been raising my other daughter's two children—but now their father took them and he says he wants them to forget that I've ever lived."

I wonder how one woman can have so much sorrow.

"But, you know, Laurel, when I get my big settlement, I bet I get my grandkids back."

CHAPTER 13

The Forever Home

January 31

Two years ago, I complained to Lyn, my trusted horoscope reader for over three decades, that I was dissatisfied with my spiritual growth. I was in a rut and what did the planets have to tell me. Lyn didn't look at her star-chart, but asked me how I felt when I came into my house. "Awful," I said. "The macadam driveway is shredding and the lawn's relentless march across it has narrowed it to barely a car's width... And my garage door doesn't want to open. And the brick-steps! They are crumbling under foot. Ernest has Quikcreted them in place, but it doesn't hold them... and there is too much distance between each step... my aging friends can't get in my house... and the house needs to be painted and I think there's some wood-rot... and, in the kitchen, the wallpaper is twenty-year-old country-boring and is peeling off the walls... and..." Lyn interrupted me, asking about my bedroom. "I hate the color of the walls—lackluster puce."

"Change your entrance, kitchen and bedroom," Lyn counseled. "And the Spiritual will follow."

Thus began eighteen months of home renovation, beginning with my phoning Karen, the only woman on Creative Paints list of painters/wallpaperers.

"I'm just up the street from you, now," Karen said. "I'll be through here in an hour. Would this be a good time to come?"

A red-haired Karen arrived in her "whites" in her red truck. Talk about the universe synchronizing my life. We took to each other immediately. She urged me to make major changes in my color palette starting in the kitchen. But the kitchen connected to the equally distressed dining room, living room, and hallways, and, looking up the stairwell, you could see the rose-trellis wallpaper of the anteroom and from there the cabbage-rose wallpapers of the guest room and coordinated striped wallpaper of the upstairs bathroom. Karen suggested we redo it all. "Doesn't that make sense?" she asked. Gone with the wallpaper, gone with the pastels! In with saturated earth colors—dark slate blue, Etruscan golds, summer's greens. All colors decided upon except the one for my bedroom.

"Do you want your bedroom dark or light?" Karen asked.

"I don't know," I said.

My art interests would now be manifested in creating beauty, not on canvas or in books—but in my living spaces. Karen and I started with the kitchen, which seemed to have a life—or should I say, death—of its own. Every appliance broke down. Stopped working. Or leaked, like the refrigerator and blender. Even the coffee bean grinder ground to a halt. Why not? They were all bought at the same time some twenty years ago.

I became my own contractor. I scoured kitchen appliance departments, searching for ones small enough to fit into our older Cape Cod-style house with its low placed cabinets and narrow spaces; I sleuthed in the tile store for multi-colored slate backsplashes and the countertop store for greenish solid-surface counters; I Googled for the particular polished nickel cabinet pulls and light switches that I desired; and I visited every lighting store in the region looking for modern glass and polished nickel light-fixtures, finally found at Lowes. My days were consumed with conferring with Karen, finding the products, finding the workers to install them, and then monitoring their work. Any tendencies I had towards obsessive-compulsiveness manifested. I had invested much of myself into the kitchen's transformation. I loved how it all looked, but my "contracting" days were over. I loved making aesthetic choices, particularly with Karen at my side giving me confidence, but I did not like administrative, managerial, bossy kind of work.

"Hire Tom Eastwood," my son Ben suggested.

Karen stayed and Tom of Cornerstone Construction came and when he had left—a year later—we had a new concrete driveway, entrances, windows, gutters, garage doors, dusty-green colored shake-siding, a black dimensional roof, re-located drains, outdoor lighting, a new electrical circuit box, recessed lights, shutters, redone wood floors, a "library" room and a new mortgage with a low interest rate.

Ernest and I have lived in this South Street house for thirty-two years. So very unlike my childhood, when Father bought houses for us to live in that he considered real-estate investments to improve and sell for a profit. I had seven different addresses before I turned eleven. Now, it was as if Ernest and I had moved into a new house without moving. Just like our Papillons, I, too, would have a forever home.

Karen and I walked around the outside of the house. "Do you love it?" she asked.

We walked around the inside. Karen had not only painted, she had rearranged the furniture, creating more open feeling spaces, and created the "library" room. From the basement, she had retrieved my carved English Tudor triangle chair and set it in a corner of the dining room. When I was five years old, Father took his three children to an antique store. The cash-poor owner chose to pay Father for his law work with furniture. Each child could choose one piece. I chose the odd, bulky, dark-wood, comfortable chair in which I could sit regally, like the princess I really was. I found it gratifying, if surprising, that my parents kept the chair through their myriad house moves until it could have a home with me. That's when I learned that its matching chair is in the Chicago Historical Museum.

"Don't you just love it?" Karen asked, admiring her handiwork.

"I do. If we only live here for a month, it's worth it!"

"What's your favorite?"

"All of it . . . maybe the dark slate blue . . . the kitchen."

"Mine, too." Karen said.

We walked upstairs. Ernest joined us.

"What about your bedroom?" Karen asked.

"I still can't decide if I want to go dark or light," I said.

"Maybe you and Ernest want to look at some paint samples? Doesn't that make sense?"

"How about this?" Ernest said, holding a saturated blue-green paint chip. "It's called 'Mountain Laurel.'"

"Perfect!" I said, making a kissing sound. "It will look light and dark. When I wake up in the morning, I'll think I'm in a thicket."

"Are you ready?" Prem asks me without the preamble of niceties about how I'm feeling and did I have a good night and am I excited. I can't help but wonder if he likes the "human" side of his p.t. job, and if he wouldn't rather be a surgeon, invisible in scrubs and face mask with a nurse or two at his side placating patients. He has long fingers, too, like surgeons are supposed to have.

"Have you ever thought about being a surgeon?" I ask, ignoring his question about my "readiness."

"Here's your jacket, Laurel," Ernest says. He hand signals me to mind my own business. Prem looks down on me. "I was a surgeon," he says. "In India."

I think I know the rest of that story. His Indian diploma does not entitle him to a surgical practice in America. Getting retrained might be just too long, costly, and demeaning.

"I'm on the waiting list in Cleveland," he says, offhandedly. "For a residency."

"Wonderful! And your family?" I ask.

Ernest shrugs his discontent about my unbridled nosiness.

"They will be back next month…So, are you ready?" Prem repeats as Ernest helps me into my wheeled walker. Today, Prem is doing the pre-discharge evaluation of my house. I will be proud to show it off. I look forward to basking in its saturated colors. "I will follow you and your husband."

"Do you mean, I'm going with Ernest? Not you?"

"Yes."

This will be the first time that Ernest will be wholly responsible for my safety and we are both surprised at this turn of events, and I am a little scared. Well, a lot scared. Something new still scares me.

More. I am frightened of being outside the protected walls of the Bellemont. I have become institutionalized—dependent on predictability, care-takers, and safe enclosure. If I feel this way after twenty-seven days, I can only imagine how disoriented and frightened a patient might feel after a long-term hospitalization, medical or mental. Leaving any total-institution is traumatic. How do released prisoners cope with the freedom? Does the prison social-worker prepare them for society? Or, is giving them back their belongings and a little money for bus fare considered ample? No wonder the high rates of recidivism.

"I can't get through the door by myself," I complain.

"I'll hold it for you," Ernest says.

"Look at how icy the walkway is," I complain.

"Your walker will give you stability," Prem says.

"I've never gotten into a sedan before," I announce, when Ernest brings my car to the awning.

"It's no different than getting into the SUV," Prem says.

Ernest folds up my walker and puts it in the backseat.

"I didn't know it would fold-up," I say. "That's nifty"

Ernest fastens my seat belt. I am anxious the whole seven minutes it takes to get to our home. I see it as we turn the corner at Evening Street: it is the handsomest house on the block. We pull onto our new concrete driveway, wide enough to be a landing strip, and Prem pulls in behind us.

"Ernest, I'll need your help getting out," I whine.

"Pivot as if you were in a regular chair," Prem instructs. "Lead out with your good foot."

Prem walks around our house inspecting its entrances like a burglar. He doesn't comment on the house's new crisp shakes. He doesn't look at me, only the house entrances and his clipboard. The front door requires walking up an uneven path to three concrete steps, the kitchen door has three steps, but the third step is small, and the back-door has three steps, but there is an uneven brick walkway getting to it.

"Can you get a ramp built?" Prem asks.

"No!" Ernest and I concur.

"Her foot problem is only temporary," Ernest says, nicely.

"Then, you'll use the kitchen door," Prem instructs.

"The storm door is very heavy and tight," I say. "And I won't be able to open it."

"Ernest, you will do that," Prem orders. "She won't be going out by herself."

And now I am invisible. Invalid. In-valid.

"And within a couple of feet there's the basement stairs," I complain. "I could fall down those."

"I'll close the folding door," Ernest says.

"Good idea." Prem concurs.

What is that parable? It is harder for a woman in a leg cast to get through the kitchen door than it is for a camel to get through a needle? Something like that.

"Yap-yap."

"Yap-yap-yap."

Bashi and Lily are going nuts in their crates.

"Don't let them out," Prem orders.

"Why?" I ask.

"They'll be in the way."

"Hi Pappies... I don't care what Prem says, you're coming out of those crates. Ernest, will you let the dogs out... I can't do it." I cannot balance myself on my walker and open the crates' doors. That's probably in the Very Advanced occupational therapy curriculum.

"Are you afraid of dogs, Prem?" I ask.

His body-language says, "Yes."

"Paws off Prem," Ernest tells the dogs. "Four on the floor." Prem begins his evaluation of the house. He doesn't notice how aesthetically pleasing everything is. Maybe he has been instructed not to comment on how a place looks, but only on what it needs for the safety of the discharged patient. Prem begins that litany. For the first floor bathroom, I will need a lift for the toilet and a twisting seat for the bath-tub. Throughout, all rugs, even the 9 x 12 ones, must be removed. I will not be allowed up the stairs to my bedroom or down the stairs to the television room. I will need a hospital bed set up in the living room with a bedside commode. My dogs will have to be crated if I am home alone—or if Ernest is busy upstairs or downstairs. I will not be able to leave the house without assistance. Any clutter on the floors, in the corners, peeking out of closets, secreted in treacherous boxes high on shelves must be attended to and, well, whatever I need in my activities of daily living should be made more accessible. And, of course, no driving.

My walker with wheels is bumping walls. The doorway into the downstairs bathroom is too narrow. I will have to enter it side-ways with my back to the toilet, if I want to use it. I burst into tears. Why would I want to come home, if so much of it has to change? Why would I want to come home when I will be so restricted? And why did I not think about modifying my house for easier access for when Ernest and I are older? Denial, that's why.

"Laurel," Ernest says. "We'll figure out the stairs."

"You can't go up." Prem is stern. "The stairs are too steep and too narrow."

I look hard at them. Mastering the physical world is not one of my strong points, but Colleen has taught me well, taught me to analyze each new situation, its constraints and possibilities.

"Yes, I can!" I glare at Prem. "If I walk duck-footed and put my good foot up first and then have my bad one join it on the stair, I can do it. One stair at a time."

I take hold of the banister and begin my ascent. Fourteen stairs. Ernest is behind me and Prem behind him. We move like a disjoint-ed dragon. I curl around the balustrade and wait for Prem to go back down and bring up my walker.

"You'll need another walker up here," he says."Medicare won't pay for it."

"Or a cane," Ernest suggests.

"A cane." I concur.

"Medicare won't pay for the cane, either," Prem says.

"How much can a cane cost?" Ernest asks. "Plus we do have Uncle Tommy's old cane here somewhere unless I've already given it away."

"You gave it to Nadia for her Halloween costume as a Ziegfeld Follies show-girl." I love this conversation, memories normalizing the abnormal.

We make our way to the upstairs bathroom which has a wider door, a walk-in shower and a raised toilet. If we bring up the shower-chair we purchased, it will work just fine. And my bed is just fine, too. Bashi and Lily jump on it.

"We're not taking a dog-nap," I say. "I'm sorry."

"You can come down once a day only," Prem commands, writing something on my chart.

I walk duck-footed down the stairs with Ernest in front, in case I should fall and Prem behind, carrying the walker.

"You can stay home for awhile, now," Prem says. He abruptly leaves by the kitchen door.

"Let's see if I can get back up the stairs," I say to Ernest.

He stands behind me as I consciously place one foot after the other on stair after stair until I reach the top. Bashi and Lily run on up and onto my bed.

On my bedroom door's doorknob is a gift from a woman I never met. She did her doctoral work in Nigeria with women building economic resources for their families. She had written me a letter that said that my writing/work had given her permission and inspiration to follow her dream. With the letter came a beautiful beaded necklace, made by the Nigerian women. "I thought these colors would look good on you," she had written. How would she have known that these are my favorite color combinations?

"Dog-nap?" I ask my pups.

"Yap."

"Yap-yap-yap."

Lily settles by my feet, Bashi makes a den from the oversized pillow.

Two hours pass. Ernest hears me stirring. He helps me to the bathroom. Waits. Helps me back to the bedroom. I'm completely dependent on him. We both fear I will fall, and that he won't be able to catch me. But I don't fall. We manage. A cause for celebration! Ernest walks ahead of me down the stairs and gives me my walker. Another cause for celebration!

Everywhere I look, I see gifts that were given to me with love. My entire house is bursting with love tokens. My body feels the vibrations. On my study's walls: The Women Prophets poster, a gift from Linda M.; a photo taken by Mr. Feenly of the Chicago Tribune at Dolly's Sixteenth Birthday party—me not yet 10, center stage, bursting with energy; a Certificate of Merit presented to my sister Jessica for her work with developmentally delayed children; on my desk, *Learning Landscapes*, a book about poetry as a research tool, dedicated to me by its editors; the desk, itself, crafted by my son Josh, and the computer put together and updated by my grandson Akiva. On the windowsill, a poured paper collage made by my friend Nan, a cartoon sent by my friend Ellyn, the human emigration map sent by Jo, and a Florida post-card from my father, sent in 1971, to my son Ben. Out my picture window, I see a circus of birds and squirrels, invited to our yard by a food buffet and a heated bird-bath, maintained by my husband Ernest.

All around me is love. *Why hadn't I noticed this before?*

February 1

"How'd your visit home go?" Colleen asks me. I can see the shape of a new back-brace under her shirt. She isn't limping any more.

"That Prem!" I say. "He tells me I can't do anything. If I listen to him, I'll be a prisoner on the first floor of my own house."

"He has to tell you about any dangers in your house as part of the discharge process. It's the law. We could be sued if you weren't informed about how to be safe at home." Colleen pauses. "But, you don't have to listen to him, and you didn't hear that from me."

"Let's practice the basement stairs," I say, thinking *I'll show him!*

"This will be your last p.t. day," Colleen says. "You can't have p.t. the day before you go home. It's another one of the laws."

I walk up and down the basement stairs three times just for good measure.

"Thanks, Colleen, for everything."

"My pleasure, Laurel."

"And best of luck in your next career! Colleen-the-Surgical-Nurse!"

"Hey girl, thanks for remembering."

"Effie Lou, how're things?"

"It's not cancer that's causin' the swelling of Tony's ball." Effie Lou turns away.

I wait for a further explanation, but Effie Lou is through talking about it. I wonder if it is something worse . . . worse for their marriage . . .

"Jes what Ah thought." Effie Lou is looking at my occupation therapy chart. "You're good to go. Y'all done done it all. Medicare is through with y'all."

"Because of you being so good!" I say.

We hug each other. I have listened to Effie Lou talk about the turmoil in her brand-new marriage. I have come to care about Effie Lou and want to know how her life story will unfold. But I realize, I do not care enough to continue our relationship once I leave. Nor do I think Effie Lou wants that either. She could talk so freely to me because she knew our relationship was time bound, limited. It was a one-way relationship. I shared nothing personal.

Effie Lou returns to her desk area. She looks heavier today than yesterday. I am hoping that all goes well for her—her health, marriage, step-son, job prospects, and dogs—and that one of her new clients is a good listener.

"How did your visit home go?" My Artist's Way young friend Tina has come for lunch bringing a gluten-free kale soup with soft tofu. She has been on a liver cleanse and her skin and soul are radiant. I think I even see a halo above her head.

"My house looks great," I say. "I napped in my own bed in my own Mountain Laurel thicket. But, I'm definitely going to need some help when I get home. I'll have a physical-therapist and home health-aide three times a week for a few weeks, but I am going to need some other kinds of help." Prem's directives about decluttering my house are rankling in my brain. He's right, of course... more right than he knows. The house's structure has been updated, now it is time to update the stuff inside it... Aha!

Tina clears our soup plates.

"I'll need a personal assistant," I say. "Can you suggest anyone?" I ask this question carefully. I wouldn't want to trap Tina into the job.

"What do you have in mind, Laurel?"

"I want to hire someone to help me declutter my stuff."

Tina stacks the soup bowls.

"Prem pointed out that for safety reasons I need to declutter and straighten up my things."

Tina wipes off the table.

"But making my home safe for my body is just a part of what I need... I need it to reflect how I am feeling inside. So much of my psyche has been cleansed while I have been here. My life is making so much more sense. This has been a liminal time for me... I am so much more at peace... and I want my belongings to reflect my Spirit."

"Hire me!" Tina says.

"Yes!" My question has worked! I did not want to insult, embarrass, or guilt-trip Tina, but oh my how I did want her as my personal assistant.

We arrange that she would keep track of her hours and that would I pay her per hour in lump sums. When the lump sum has been dispersed, we would revisit our agreement. Was the pay adequate? Was the working together working?

The message on Tina's phone is, "Have a joyful day!" and, I imagine, we will have many of them. I imagine myself resting on my bed while we sort through my clothes closet, relegating many to Goodwill. I imagine my clothes arranged by categories—jackets, long-sleeve shirts, short sleeve shirts, camis, pants, skirts, dresses—and color sorted within the categories. From my bed, I will see the order and the beauty of my wardrobe. Tina will have swept away the detritus on the floor and walls, and cleansed it with a sage brush and the healing sound of my reverberating Tibetan bells.

Then, there is the linen closet so full sheets, blankets and towels that the doors will not close and Ernest and I can't find within it a wash cloth or a towel. The white cotton sheets are for double beds, a size too small. How perfect they will be for Tina's massage table. The blankets and beach towels, which we never use, will bring comfort to some pre-schoolers when Tina brings them to her work-place. Once we've organized into bins the washcloths, towels, and our sheets, we'll be able to find what we want with ease.

My mind's eye browses through my books. Surely, I have sixteen boxes or so of postmodernist books that I am so through with! They can go to the University library. Novels, histories, and biographies can go to the public library. Travel books can go to the pre-school. Poetry books will stay on their shelves. Books I've made or altered will stay, too.

Then there is my studio. A world of goodies to pass on . . . card-board and mat boards to the collage group; fat-quarter quilting cloth to the Art Quilt Alliance; *Doll Magazines* to the Worthington Historical Museum; and paper, crayons, containers, boxes and gift bags and what-ever weird stuff Tina thinks might be of interest to the preschoolers or their teachers will be out of my room and into their school. What is left will be organized and shelved.

"Tina," I say. "I think we'll be sorting and organizing for over a year! I want to purge my life of that which no longer supports it or has meaning."

"This place gives me the creeps," Josh says, as he settles into a stur-dy chair at the Bellemont. He and Akiva are here for their twice-weekly visit. They never take their jackets off.

"I've only been here for a month," I say. "And I leave on Saturday."

"You are not young. Mom, and your being in here makes me think of you being here long term."

"Don't worry," I say. "That's not going to happen to me." I think he really is thinking about me dying. I'm glad he waited until I was leaving here to tell me his feelings.

"Thinking about it—the reality of seeing you here—I finally figured out why it has been so hard for me to concentrate this month. Why my school work has suffered."

"A problem for you, too, Akiva?" I ask.

"No, not really," he says, looking down. His maternal grandmother died a year ago and I am not sure he has processed that loss. He raises his head and brightens. "I have a new cello piece. Faure's *Elegy*."

I am delighted that Akiva is sharing this news.

"Do you want to hear it?"

I nod my yes.

Akiva opens Yo Yo Ma's rendition on my laptop. I see an intensity in Akiva's eyes that I haven't been privy to because I've never seen him face-on listening to music. It's as though he has been transported into a sacred space, as though he is no longer in his body in a chair in this room with his father and grandmother.

"His cello teacher has been after him all year to get a better cello," Josh says.

Akiva turns off the music—as if talking during it is a sacrilege.

"She thinks I need a better cello," Akiva says *sotto voce*.

"Do you *want* one?" Josh asks. "It means you are committed to practicing."

Akiva whispers, "I *would* like it."

"I'll go cello shopping with you when I get out of here," I announce. "What a joy that will be."

"Mom," Josh says. "Do you remember going guitar shopping with me, when I was seventeen—Akiva's age?"

"I do."

"It brought me out of my depression," Josh continues. "I told myself I would be playing it for two decades…that I'd be alive for two decades."

"And you still play, it." Akiva chimes in. "And you love it."

In two decades, I will probably not be on this earth to hear Josh playing the guitar or Akiva playing the cello—but the music will play on, and maybe I'll be in tune with the energy, as I am now.

"In two decades," Akiva says, "I will be loving and playing my cello and telling my son about his great-grandmother."

For the past month, vulnerable and fragile, I have been waited on, visited, dog-napped with, read to by Ernest, given physical therapy. Life in rehab has been exceedingly positive through the kindnesses of family, friends, and strangers—staff. I have not been treated as if I had been bad. During this sojourn, I have not been punished. I have not been abandoned.

So, how might I best spend whatever time I have left on this earth in my rehabilitated body and soul? What matters? Sitting side-by-side in front of me—my son and grandson—I know the answer: Legacy and Joy.

Nurture a child, plant a tree, write a book. Be kind. Mother's voice.

Leave the world better than you found it. Be kind. Father's voice.

Josh and Akiva lean over to give me good-by hugs and as usual high tail it down the corridor.

CHECK HALL 100 EXIT CHECK HALL 100 EXIT CHECK HALL 100 EXIT RRRRRRRRIIIIINNNNNNGGGGGG RRRRRRRRIIIIINNNNNNGGGGGG

"Hi Renee." She's in her bed. Her food tray looks as untouched as mine. "I've brought you an ice-cream drumstick."

"Come on in, Laurel," she says. Her silk flowers still look like silk flowers.

"My debriefers have been calling me," she says. "On my home-phone. Duh. And they've been calling my daughter . . . what does she know? . . . and now they're calling my cell-phone. They asked me if my cell-phone was a secure line. 'Sure,' I said. Duh! Just like all cell-phones." She starts to laugh. "I had them going there for awhile."

I laugh, too, and ask, "What do they want?"

"Because of my top security clearance, two of them have to exit-interview me at the same time. Find out what I know. Find out if they can trust me. Or if they'll have to incarcerate me or off me."

I think Renee's serious.

"They do that, you know." She winks and looks around her room. "They need a secure place to do the interview. Like, how are they going to do that here at the Bellemont?" Renee is gleeful at the prospect. "They'd have to rewire the whole place—kick everyone out of here—even you, Laurel—maybe especially you, because I've spent time with you."

"Or, maybe they could just bring a secure van into the parking lot?" I've gotten into the thriller-mode.

Renee looks at me like I'm the dumbest cube in the ice-tray. "You don't know anything about security, do you Laurel?"

"Not much. Just what I see on TV."

"That's crap. There's no way to make a van secure enough. They want me to come into the office! I'm not going to do that. Have everyone see me."

I nod my agreement and say, "That's nervy of them."

"Have you noticed the grunting woman who positions herself outside your door, across from my door?"

"I can't miss her," I say.

"She's my supervisor's mother so, maybe she doesn't really have to be here, but she's here spying on me."

"Yeah, and her grunting covers up her electronic beeper telling *them* that she hears you."

"And maybe she's got special X-ray vision glasses behind her glasses. We *have* those you know."

"And that Trevor! He acts like he's out-of-it, but have you noticed how he sometimes isn't?" I add. I'm having a blast.

"And you know about that German Frau Ilsa? I am sure there isn't anything really wrong with her. She's a trained story-teller. I can tell. I know she is a spy."

"And what about that husband of hers? He looks like military to me?" I say.

"He's CIA. I can tell. He's black and smart. I can tell."

"What do you think about Edna and that Golden Bear motif?" I ask.

"Now, that's a lie if I ever heard one! Edna broke her hip at the gym? My ass she did."

Renee does a little fist jabbing. "And I think the manager has told those Sierra Leonies to torture me until I tell them what I know but I won't break."

I am on a thriller roll and I'm laughing. At this moment, I think Renee and I could possibly be friends. She is smart, witty, and I've shared my laughing, for me more sacred than the sharing of bread.

"You can't trust anyone, Laurel." Renee turns her turtley-looking head from side-to-side. "Maybe I can't trust you? Can I? Are you wired? Are you setting me up? Is Lily part of the scheme?" She isn't smiling.

"Do you see those hundred angels dancing on the head of your light bulb?" I ask, trying to divert her.

"No-o-o." Her eyes seem to flicker.

"I guess I'll get back to my room," I say.

"Okay. Oh, thanks for the ice-cream." She coughs. "It wasn't poisoned, was it?"

Is she kidding?

February 2

"Good morning, Laurel." Brandon looks snappy today, as usual. He is carrying a half dozen large canvas bags with the Bellemont printed on them. "These are for your belongings. They're for you." He sets the bags on the floor behind the table. "Is there anything else you need?"

"You've been great," I say. "But I keep wondering about Renee."

"That's being taken care of," he says. "Anything else?"

"Did you find out what room Bingo Beth is in?"

"Sorry, I couldn't find any Beths in our system. Maybe it's a middle-name or nickname?"

"Would you give this wedding card to Brooke?" I ask. I had written a little thank-you note and enclosed a small check designated as a wedding present. I don't know if the rules prohibit tipping the staff.

Brandon puts the card into his jacket pocket.

"I haven't seen Jamal for awhile, either. Would you give him my good-byes?"

"Jamal isn't working here anymore," Brandon says.

"Good. So, he's going back to school? Do you know what major?"

"I can't talk about personnel." Talkative Brandon has clammed up.

I feel let down, not just because I don't know what happens next in Jamal's life, but because I liked him, liked talking to him about novels, and liked watching him pad around my room like a declawed cat. I thought I was playing a significant role in his recovering from flunking out of pre-med. I thought I'd edged him into finding a career. Finding himself. How hubristic of me. How Lady Bountiful-ish.

"Thanks Brandon," I say. "For all you have done. Can you give a special thanks to Gunther for me? He was a great fixer-upper."

"Yes, I can do that."

I am a rehabilitated patient and I am leaving the Bellemont, but so are many of the staff: Colleen to be a surgical nurse, Rhonda to be an athletic trainer, Brandon whenever he can, Effie Lou if the new job comes through, Jamal for some mysterious reason, Brooke likely choosing to take care of her mother, Gunther retiring soon to work on his church's fellowship hall. And, when the Bellemont gets purchased by a national residential care firm, which I am sure will happen, most, if not all, of the administrative staff will be looking for work elsewhere. *Good Luck!*

Ring-ring.

"Hello."

"Hello, Miss Richardson." Johnetta's voice. "You need to come to the Therapy Room and sign your discharge papers. Is this a good time?"

"Perfect!"

Johnetta is waiting for me at the Therapy Room door. I follow her into a large office with a messy desk. On the left side of the desk there is a little clearing. In it there is a silver picture frame holding a photo of a dressed-up smiling little girl. The photo is probably always in Johnetta's line of sight.

"What a cute girl," I say.

"Thanks." Johnetta smiles at the photo. "She is very smart, too." Johnetta pushes paper at me to sign, and explains the discharge process in bureaucraticese.

"Can you explain that again," I ask.

"This is today."

"Yes." I say. *I do know that.* "The day before I leave."

"According to Medicare Rules—here's the page." She shows me a print-out in Times Roman font size 8—maybe 6.

"I can't read that," I say, squinting.

Johnetta reads. "If you think you're being asked to leave or to be discharged too soon, you may have the right to ask for a review of the discharge decision by an independent reviewer called a Quality Improvement Organization (QIO) before you leave." She points to the page. "Do you understand?"

"I do. And, I am ready to go home tomorrow."

"Not tomorrow," Johnetta announces.

"What? Why?"

"Medicare rule. The facility has to give you two-days notice."

"Then, why didn't you give me notice yesterday?" I am angry.

"Your paperwork wasn't finished."

"Who does the paperwork?"

"I do." Johnetta says. "You don't have to stay the extra day, though. We can't make you stay."

"Okay. I am leaving tomorrow."

I walk my walker into the corridor.

Jingle-jangle.
"Yap-Yap-Yap."

"Hi, Lily . . . Hi, Bashi . . . my beautiful little dogs."

Bashi wags his tail. Lily sits, waiting to be picked up.

I give Ernest a kiss and tell him about my interview with Johnetta, concluding with," I wonder how much extra money the nursing home makes from Medicare for residents who aren't there."

"Yesterday upon the stair, I met a man who wasn't there," Ernest starts reciting.

"He wasn't there again today," I add.

"I wish that man would go away."

"Li lee Li lee Li lee." Trevor is shouting.

"Sweet little puppy-doodle-bugs," Edna is calling my dogs.

"Hi, Edna." I say. I encourage the dogs to keep walking.

"Grunt . . . Cha . . . Cha . . . " The Corridor Woman is near my door. The dogs ignore her.

"Lily, come see me." Renee says. Ernest puts Lily on Renee's lap.

"Lily's claws are hurting me," Renee says.

"I'll take her." Ernest says.

Renee snap-wheels herself back into her room and slams her door.

"Yap-yap-yap."

"Dogs. This is your last time on my bed, here." I look them square in their eyes. "What do you think of that?"

"Yap-yappity-yap-yap!"

I think that means, hip-hip-hooray."

Three of my Artist Way friends have arrived for a going-home celebratory lunch. Carol brings placemats, flowers and a salad; Tina, kale soup and crackers; and Jo, cookies and silvery head bands for each one of us. Of course, we look adorable in them. Well, festive anyway. I have brought nothing, other than an ethical question that I am eager to discuss with them: How do I terminate my relationship with Renee?

Renee considers me her only friend. I've listened to her medical, legal, emotional, and familial problems. I've built a relationship with her. I feel compassion for her losses—legs, job, independence, sense of being attractive, and possibly her home and grandchildren. I admire her guts and survival skills. But, she is obsessed with getting Lily, and she may well have access to nefarious ways of doing so. And for now, at least, she has added me to her paranoiac panoply of bad guys.

"Simply wish her well, before you leave." Jo advises. "Thank her for helping Lily become a therapy dog."

"Write her a letter, *after you've* left." Tina advises.

"Trust yourself and the universe," Carol says. "It'll work out."

None of them advises me to give Renee a false phone-number and address, or to give her false hopes of a continuing relationship. Each of them has heard me.

"Shall I lead us in a meditation?" Tina asks.

We nod our assent.

"Close your eyes," Tina says. "Breathe deeply . . . Imagine that you are in a safe place—and that five years from now have passed . . . Where are you? . . . Who is with you? . . . What are you doing? . . . What do you need? . . . Want?"

I go deep into myself.

"Open your eyes," Tina says. "Come back to here and now . . . Anyone want to talk about their experience?"

"Oh, I do!" I say. "I am at a beach. Surrounding me are all my friends from all the times in my life, and, like the Hopi Story-Telling Kachina, all around me little children and babies run and jump and play. Everything I need I already have. I long for nothing."

I long for nothing.

After my Artist Way friends leave, I find myself wondering where the people I've met at the Bellemont will be in five years. I will probably never see them again, but I care about them and feel gratitude toward them. Each one of them—knowingly or not—has contributed to my physical and emotional rehabilitation—not just from ankle surgery, but from a lifetime of a self-blaming narrative. Each one—I think—is like the apocryphal butterfly whose fluttering wings is felt in unexpected places.

Ring. Ring.

"Hi, Mom." Ben's voice.

"Hi, Laurel." Tami's voice.

Their phone is on speaker.

"How're you doing?" Ben asks.

"Going home tomorrow," I say.

"Anything we can do for you?" Tami asks.

"Bashi and Lily would love for you to visit." I say.

At five, Ernest comes in without the dogs. "How about supper at the Thai place and a visit home?" Ernest suggests. This is to be my last night at the Bellemont, and an outing sounds particularly good because I will be housebound after I leave. "We can take some of your stuff home too." I look at how little I have brought with me. For a month, I have done just fine with a limited wardrobe, a laptop, a couple of books, dog-treats, dopp-kit: I've been in boot-camp in preparation for my house-decluttering.

Leftovers in a smartly folded carryout bag attach to my walker, and with Ernest leading the way, we come into our "new-old" home. Lily and Bashi are yapping me a welcome. On the kitchen table, there are greeting cards:

A barefooted little farm-girl against a dark barn getting kisses from the dog on her lap signed, XO.

A little house with a white-picket fence and a rainbow over its roof. Glad to hear you're back home, Love, Elaine

A Parisian scene and long note from Pat.

A postcard from Hawaii from Bev.

And on the table a bouquet of lavender lilies, magenta carnations, baby's breath and lush greens sent all the way from Australia—well, ordered from there anyway—from my dear friend, Julie. "Glad you're home, Laurel, and hope these bring some cheer."

"Tomorrow . . . tomorrow!" I sing out Little Orphan Annie's song.

Renee's door is open when I get back to the Bellemont. I peek in.

"Going home to your pool tomorrow, huh, Laurel?" Renee has a wry smile on her face.

"You know I don't have a pool," I say, my arms akimbo at my hips.

"But you are going home."

"Yes."

"I'm getting kicked out," Renee announces. "That Rhonda says I am not progressing enough. My father is looking into other places for me. Ones closer to him. I think all the staff want me gone. I'm too much trouble."

"I'm sorry, Renee."

"Here's my phone number." Renee tears off a little corner of the daily menu and writes her number on it in pencil."

I put the little piece in the kangaroo pocket of my hoodie. She doesn't ask for my phone number. I am grateful that Renee is making this easy for me. Maybe she doesn't want to keep the relationship going either?

"I'll miss Lily," she says.

"I'll try to bring her tomorrow before I leave."

We do not hug.

We have never touched one another.

I dream I am on a dark stage on a love-seat with a man I can't quite identify. It might be my special colleague Clyde, an African American gay man from Memphis, who died too young. Or maybe it's Jamal— or maybe it's my husband Ernest—or my animus. The curtains have parted and the man and I are filling the theater with our exuberance, laughter and playfulness. We look at each other, and together shout-out, "Kisses in the dark!" The audience cheers.

February 3

"Good morning, Laurel." A baritone voice. the Bellemont's' Dr. Miller is standing at the foot of my bed. His blond nurse Kathy is standing beside him. It is 5:30 in the morning. *Déjà vu.*

"So, you are being discharged today," Dr. Miller says. "How do you feel?"

"Good," I say.

"Any pain?"

"Just a little at my big toe joint."

"I can't see it through your cast," he says, chortling.

I smile.

"Kathy, write a prescription for Laurel for Oxycodone."

"I don't want it," I say.

"Yes, of course… You want the new one… Opana."

"No!" I say.

"Okay… Kathy, write it for Vicodin."

"No, I don't want any pain pills."

"But you might need them when you get home… Kathy can phone in the order."

"I don't want them!" I repeat.

Dr. Miller looks miffed. I am probably the only patient he has discharged who has refused street-ready-to-sell drugs. He listens to my heart, pounds my chest, reviews my pre-op prescriptions and pronounces me medically sound. It is 5:35 a.m.

Knock-knock.

It is 7:00. An aide I do not recognize has brought me my breakfast tray.

Jingle-jangle.

"Yap-yap."

Ernest has arrived. It is 9:00. We pack up my DonJoy cooler, Dry-Pro, clothes, and books into the Bellemont's bags. Brandon comes in at 9:30. "Here's your discharge papers," he says. "You'll have to do a final sign-out at the nurses' desk."

I scan the papers. "Look here," I say to Ernest. "Johnetta has checked that I am of *average* intelligence."

"I'll tell the manager, Thomas, that you're ready to leave," Brandon says. "He'll want to say good-bye to you. He's in Renee's room right now. I'll get him"

"Thank you for doing your recovery with us," Thomas-the-manager says. He is not wearing a tie or suit-jacket. I have seen him before in the hallways, but I thought he was a family member. We had exchanged greetings, but had never been introduced.

"So, you are the one who lent me your scooter," I say. "Thanks."

"I'm glad it was useful," Thomas says. "And, again, thank you for having chosen the Bellemont." He dips back into Renee's room. I can see her on the bed. She waves a little high-five good-bye. Thomas closes her door.

"I'll carry your things out," Brandon says, slipping the bags over his shoulders.

"Thanks again for everything, Brandon, "I say. "And good luck."

Ernest and I stop at the nurses' desk where Ernest signs me permanently out.

"Hi," Trevor says.

"Bye, Trevor," I say.

"Yap."

"Yap."

"Bye bye dogs." Trevor says.

I look into the Therapy Room and blow kisses to Colleen and Effie Lou.

Kisses in the light.

February 4

I dreamt last night that all manner of warfare and mayhem is going on around me. Invaders. Marauding troops. Destruction all around. Whole cities being evacuated. Peoples migrating. I can't find Ernest. I don't know if he has decided to migrate or not. I am alone. I decide to stay just where I am.

CHAPTER 14

Temporarily Abled

November 5

Ten months have passed since my ankle surgery. My home health-care helpers have come and gone. My Prussian-blue foot cast is gone, replaced for six months with a black walking-boot, which is gone now, too, replaced with Nikes, Kinesia tapes, and orthotics. Six months of outpatient physical therapy is over. A month ago, I could feel the ground with my left foot for the first time. Two days later, my left foot felt heavy, the numbness at last gone. The cane, walker, and shower chair are stowed in the basement whose stairs I can go down and up. I have no fear of falling.

Our Papillons, Bashi and Lily, having turned three, are now considered adult dogs. Lily has qualified as a Canine Good Citizen and Bashi is but a bark away from that certification. We are waiting for their therapy dog certification tests. They will resume dog agility training next month. Two weeks ago, they accompanied Ernest and me to our time-share in Sedona, where we all hiked on Deer Pass Trail.

My family's good. My grandson Akiva has a new/old cello, passed his GED, and started college. Dialysis has revitalized my brother-in law. He'll turn 85 in two months. He's treating his lady-friend to skydiving lessons and leading his continuing care community's fight against their new management's food policies. I sent him a Happy Halloween card. My brother will be getting both hips replaced in January. My cousin Barbara continues to shun me for having written about her family. Rarely do I lose one person at a time. Rather, my losses are of whole groups like my sociology department when I retired, the Bellemont people when I left, and, now more painful, following Barbara's lead, all my gentile relatives are incommunicado.

My house has gone through its first round of decluttering with my friend Tina doing the hard labor and coaching. It is quiet and easy here in my home. It is if all that I have learned while in the Bellemont is settling into me: Continuing to heal body and spirit.

I have had the luxury of time to recover from my fall and surgery, to think about my experience as person with a visible disability, and to read about others' experiences and our social and cultural responses. The issues are multilayered and complex: the proverbial elephant is in the room. It is surrounded by engaged and smart viewers. Each viewer focuses on something different, a patch of skin, a crease in the trunk, a flick of the tail. It is not that any of the viewers are wrong, it is just that the *whole* elephant is really BIG—and does not stand still or forget . . . and that the viewers, themselves, are moving about.

My thoughts are moving, too, as I view the viewers of the elephant. Most look through the lenses that divide nature from culture, just as poets and philosophers have done for centuries. So, the elephant is seen as a either a social *construction* or an *embodiment*.

The unsettledness and excitement I felt when thinking about cyborgs, a material example of the leakiness in the boundary between *nature* and *culture* returns. Maybe I can alter the visions of the elephant's viewers by blurring boundaries? And maybe by so doing both the rehabilitation system and the individuals it serves will profit.

I can make a little step forward. But first I will have to back-up and talk some about the tenets of social *constructionism*. It holds that the way we *see* the world is inherited from those who came before us and is learned through social-interaction. We reinforce that inherited world by our actions and pass it on to our progeny. How we interact with each other becomes institutionalized. We come to *believe* that what we do is the natural and right way. We make meaning. For example, we invest gold, not gravel, with value. We *buy* dogs, and then call them *family*. When we see a Top Doc plaque on our surgeon's wall, we hunker down and invent *good* reasons why we are waiting so long in the waiting room. The meanings we make are always contextual, influenced by the time and spaces in which we are living. Meaning does not rest in objects. We put meaning into the objects. Everything that humans do or make is socially constructed. This includes all of our categories, evaluations thereof, and language, itself. Because humans have made it, they can—and do—remake it. Rather than searching for the *truth*, then, a social constructionist is interested in how the claim to truth is constructed and *who benefits.*

Social constructionists have applied these tenets to our ideas about gender and race. *Gender* is viewed as *performed*—accomplished through social interactions, actual or imagined. Gender is not what one *is*, but what one *does* to convince oneself and others that one is a male (such as keeping on beard stubble, wearing falling-down jeans with chain belts and untied Air Jordan high-tops, sitting with legs spread) or female (such as putting on make-up, wearing tummy-revealing T-shirts and glitzy sandals, sitting with legs crossed). Sometimes, when window shopping at the mall, I hear an angry sounding question about a fellow shopper: "Is *that* a boy or a girl?" The window shopper's uncategorizeable gender performance underscores the expectation for the familiar and the latent anger that underlies seeing it violated. By social decree, there are only two mutually exclusive gender categories. But, it is not just at leisure, getting dressed and shopping the mall, where gender matters. Gender is an *omnirelevant* category, always at play, always shaping social and legal institutions and economic consequences. Even those men who would have it differently, enjoy the male privileges of higher status, greater earning power, and control of governmental decision-making.

Race is another social construction that is omnirelevant, affecting our everyday lives and social institutions. Race does not exist in any *objective* way—that is there are no objective markers that can categorize people as say, black or white. There are biological overlaps. But *race* as a concept is very real in society, shaping the way we see ourselves and others, and creating institutions that are steeped in racism. Dominant groups act as if there is a biological reality that justifies creating boundaries that exclude those of a race deemed lesser. In America, following the civil war, skin color became the marker. It still is. Racism continues to work because a racialized society exists in which whites are blind to the everyday and institutional benefits proffered to them because of their skin color.

Gender and race, then, as social constructions, depend upon collective acceptance and agreement. The dominant group—whether it be men in reference to women, or whites in reference to blacks—sets the rules, agenda, ideology that includes or excludes, disables or enables power. There are shelves and shelves of books that address the problems of sexism and racism.

Time now to raise another omnirelevant "ism": *Ableism.* Like gender and race, able-ness is socially constructed as consisting of two poles—*ability* or *disability.* Like gender and race, the dominant—the able-bodied—control the rules, agenda, and ideology. In common parlance and medical-talk, one either is or is not disabled. And, in the same way that gender and race shape all our lives, so does the idea of disability.

Having a disability is part of the human condition. How it is received and treated varies by time and culture. Our Western culture inherited the Greek consciousness of the philosopher Aristotle. In *Politics* he wrote, "Let there be a law that no deformed child should live." Such children were routinely exposed to inclement weather. With the rise of Christianity, the routine practice of infanticide was replaced with other practices: church shelters, separate towns and colonies for the disabled, shipping them off to faraway ports where they would languish to death—or, putting them in "idiot cages" in public squares where townspeople could laugh and taunt.

In the mid-nineteenth century, a new consciousness entered Europe. Arising out of what was called "political arithmetic," what we now call *statistics,* was the idea of the *normal.* The "normal bell-shaped curve" was held not only to *describe* the variations in human heights, weights, head circumferences and so on, it conferred upon the *average* measurements a special status. Both progressive and reactionary activists proposed eugenics programs through which deviations from the mean would diminish and defects of the body would disappear. With the idea of the norm, came the idea of the *deviant*—bodies lying outside the *normal* curve. Any thoughts we have about *normalcy* are inexorably tied to ideas about *deviance*.

When a temporarily abled person sees someone who is limbless, wheelchair-bound, palsied, or otherwise physically marked, they see deviance from *normalcy* and label that person as *disabled*. A boy's stare at a girl's thalidomide-affected foreshortened arms, his mother telling him not to stare while she herself does exactly that, her face registering pity, pain, repulsion, and fear, is a social-interaction I experienced when taking care of a friend's daughter. I thought, *Does that woman not know that I can see that she is staring exactly like her son and that I can see the emotions on her face?* One of my friends chose not to visit me at the Bellemont because she "can't stand seeing *those* people warehoused there." A middle-aged woman looks away, speeds up, after she sees my bent-over arthritic friend and me sitting at the outdoor café. I feel the anger mounting in the queue behind me when a man on crutches in front of me is a very *slow* man. A Yorkie dog breeder refuses to sell a puppy to my friend with Parkinson's. A clutch of neighbors complain about their tax dollars being used to install wheelchair-friendly curbs. They are openly odious in their speech. A property manager acquaintance won't rent to the physically disabled because they might, she says, fall and sue, or fall and damage the property, or not keep it clean, or have friends like themselves who will fall and sue. She is legally allowed to refuse renting to disabled people, she says, as long as she does not give their disability as the reason. My neighbor Renee at the Bellemont was stripped of her high security clearance and fired from her Energy Department consulting job after losing her legs—not her mind.

From casual interactions, to the ownership of pets to walking about, making a living and finding a place to live, one's apparent *normalcy* gives one privileges—just like being male and white do. But the social construction of disability goes even further than that of gender and race because disability is constructed as a *totalizing* entity, as something that takes over the person and defines them. One can be a black woman writer and be invested and accepted in all three identities. But blind and deaf Helen Keller becomes a poster-child for courage in overcoming her disability. Her life-long activism in socialist causes and the free love movement are erased. The physical challenges of people such as Rosa Luxemborg (who limped), Antonio Gransci (crippled, dwarf hunchback), Alexander Pope (dwarfed hunchback), Byron (club foot), Harriet Martineau (deaf), Frido Kahlo (osteomyelitis), and Virginia Woolf (lupus) are usually ignored. Because they have created canonical works, they are assumed to be physically able. In our commonplace thinking—unless one is an *extremely extreme* exception, such as Stephen Hawking—one cannot be *disabled* and *able*. Even President Franklin Delano Roosevelt was not photographed in his wheelchair.

Societal beliefs are created, maintained, and handed down through the generations. Different ideas become linked. In the history of our social construction of disability, *physical* disability has been conflated with *moral depravity.* Over one hundred thousand residents of institutions for the mentally and physically disabled in America have been buried without names on their gravestones, as a kindness to their families to protect them from stigma and shame. My father passed on to me the idea that to be disabled is to be bad through the cloak of his incipient Christian Science. Some New Age and other religious practitioners inculcate their flocks with that belief, too. Some sermonize that disabledness is the mark of Satan.

The nineteenth-century forensic physician Cesare Lombroso claimed that criminals could be differentiated from law-abiding people by distinguishing facial and bodily characteristics, such as long arms and asymmetry. In the twentieth century, persons of power and influence, such as Prime Ministers Churchill and Chamberlin, President Theodore Roosevelt. John Rockefeller, H.G. Wells, Maynard Keynes and, especially noteworthy, the "Mother" of birth control, Margaret Sanger, were active in the eugenics movement. It held that if eugenics knowledge was instituted the world would be free of the defective, diseased, crippled and depraved. Not that long ago—in 1933—the prominent science journal, *Nature,* approved the Nazi's proposal to sterilize those with congenital infirmities of body or mind. Hitler's policies grew out of American and English eugenics. The first to be murdered by Hitler were the "useless eaters," the "life unworthy of life"—that is, *the disabled.* Two hundred thousand were "mercy killed." Medical doctors were the executioners.

When I was a college sophomore, I was a summer hire in Cook County's welfare system. My caseload was young women with physical and mental limitations. I was instructed to convince them to get sterilized "for their own good and the good of the city." Babies they might have, I was told, would drain our meager resources. The boys would probably be thieves and rapists ending up in prison and the girls would end up on the streets as prostitutes. I did not follow my orders; my summer employment was terminated. This was in the late 1950s.

Lombroso's claim has been disproved and the eugenics movement is at bay, although it continues to live in selective abortion, genetic counseling, and in some bioethicists. Peter Singer, the bioethics chair at Princeton University and winner of several bioethics awards has written that, "Killing a disabled baby is not the moral equivalent of killing a person." But, the killing should be done in the first month of the baby's life. Singer is the founder of the animal rights movement.

Selective abortion is the new way of enacting eugenics. Some children—because of disabilities seeable or measureable pre-birth—are unworthy of life or will be troublesome and expensive should they be born. Friends of mine are parents of a daughter, Oma, with tuberous sclerosis (TS), a hereditary condition in which the nerves are not completely sheathed. She has facial stigmata, inoperable brain tumors, kidney dysfunction, an uneven gait and seizures. She is also a PhD in French Literature, a wife, and a step-mother of three. Oma was diagnosed when she was three years old, her mother four months pregnant with another baby. The genetic counselor said the fetus had a 50% chance of having TS. *Abortion is legal,* he said. Oma's mother chose to carry the fetus to term. That second-born girl is finishing her Master's degree in—yes—genetic counseling.

The conflation of physical disability and moral depravity thrives in our popular culture. Consider the iconic images of Frankenstein, Dracula, the Joker, Dr. Strangelove, and the Phantom of the Opera—as well as the cultural morass of books, boy bands, and bricolage. Note how the Evil Villain is *physically* marked. Not only do the non-normative have to deal with our horrendous eugenics historical legacy, they live in a world where they are stigmatized anew, at psychological risk whenever they turn on the television, go to a movie, or open a book. On the brighter side, they probably can go to state fairs and circuses where side-shows of human anomalies have been eliminated.

And the *disabled* are not the only ones who are affected by our culture's social construction of disability. *Everyone* is, because everyone is only *temporarily* able-bodied. In time, through age or accident or disease or genes, everyone becomes disabled in some way. COPD changed my best friend Betty from a woman who mastered the Grand Canyon's Bright Angel Trail to one who walked hunched over, tethered to a portable oxygen tank, resting every five-steps or so on the way to the bench in her backyard. The last months of her life she spent in a hospital bed and wheelchair, no longer going outside. Being seen in a wheelchair, she felt, diminished her self-respect, pride, and self-esteem. She defined herself as *elderly* rather than *disabled.* She was only 65. "All I have left," she said, "is my dignity." To the end of her life she embraced the ideology of ableism, acting out the culture's position that to be *disabled* is to lack seemliness.

And those who are already *differently abled* will have other kinds of disabilities thrust on them. Not one thing after another but one thing on top of another. Plastic surgery and cosmetics can only stave off the appearance of aging for a while, and can do nothing to stop the internal process. Knee and hip replacements and ankle surgery can give back, for a time, the step of youth, but then, there is the other knee, hip, ankle. Looking old or odd, moving slowly or oddly on foot, with cane or not, sitting slumped or rigid in a wheelchair or not, head cocked to hear better, eyesight compromised, skin crepey.

Everyone is subject to denigration and stigmatization. Exits? Isolation or death.

I have just experienced being a person with a mobility disability, in my case a temporary non–life-threatening one. My friends face similar issues of adjusting to their aging bodies. We avoid calling ourselves *disabled* or even *people with disabilities*. "Physically challenged" are the words, often said with a smile and a wink, as if the euphemism will erase the bodily reality.

As I continue aging, one of the conversations I have with myself are "What will I do *if*?" I create ascending plans: Plan A…Plan B….Plan C. So, what happens when I no longer trust myself to drive? Plan A: Let Ernest do it. And when Ernest can't? Plan B: Ask my children to help. And, if they can't? Call on friends. And what next? Take a taxi. And, if that's too expensive? Call Senior Services. And if there aren't any? I don't want to even think about that. Indeed, I don't. In the mail today came a hand addressed invitation to a seminar hosted by Friendship Village, a continuing care community. Have I thought about what I might need in the (near) future, where I might want to live, what services I will require? These questions implicitly asked. I know I want to stay in my own home. I refuse to think I may have to leave it. I'll live in denial. I tossed the invitation into my kitchen's garbage can. My guess is there will be more invitations. And, I may have to accept one…some day. But not today.

Yet, there is a positive and hopeful side to all this. Social constructionists understand that just because something is a certain way doesn't mean it has to stay that way. They know that what humans create humans can change. Every social institution is a possible target. As the baby-boomers surge into their older age, they can be a force for change, just as they have been throughout their lives. They were the demographic force behind the civil rights, women's and gay rights social movements. Now they have aging and disability to act on. They are experienced agents of social change. They know how to lobby social and political institutions to adapt to their burgeoning population with physical and mental challenges. Buildings, public access, public transportation, design of vehicles, design of everyday objects, the material world could be remade.

A good place for all of us to start is with our verbal and nonverbal language. We no longer accept racial or gender slurs. Some of those slurs we've recuperated: *black is beautiful,* homosexuals are *queer,* ladies are *women.* Some in the *disability cultures* call themselves *crips.* Time has come for a deep and wide critical review of our signifiers, images, and metaphors regarding the "disabled." For example, we might begin by rejecting the social construction of *disability,* replacing it with the concept of *differentially abled* or preferably, *person with a disability.* We did that with AIDS. We altered our society's vision of AIDS from being a *totalizing* identity to a part of a person's life, a *person with AIDS.* We need a similar change in our consciousness about Ableism.

One way to change consciousness is to listen to those who speak from *embodiment*—not about the *theory* of the body which is so popular in the academy, but a *speaking,* if you will, from the body, what some have called the *embodied experience.*

For those in *physically challenged* bodies, *marginality* is not just a concept in postmodern criticism; it is a place their bodies occupy: on the sidelines, hugging the wall. Nancy Mairs writes about being in her wheelchair in a hotel hallway when fourteen-hundred workshoppers exited a program honoring the Dalai Lama. "And let me tell you," Mairs writes, "no matter how persuaded they were of the beauty and sacredness of all life, not one of them seemed to think that any life was going on below the level of her or his own gaze." She was pummeled on all sides by bellies and buttocks. " 'Down here!" she said. 'There's a person down here!' " Her solution? ". . . roll to one side and hug a wall."

A Paralympian, Danielle Peers, writes about the many times she has had her body and disability interrogated by medical personnel, disability experts, geneticists, Paralympian sport classifiers who give "handicap" ratings to the athletes, and *normates.* She writes about the process through which she is not just called *disabled,* but willingly confesses to it, holds it to be true, preferring the tap-tap-tapping of a cane to the smack of shod feet against the wooden floor, welcomes the *wheelers* and *crutchers* who compete in her sport. Being aware that she might be watched and judged by both normates and Paralympic competitors, she watches, judges and disciplines herself. She doesn't want to look too disabled in public, and she doesn't want to look too able in her sport lest she be called a *cheater*. Mostly, she wants to re-write the cultural story, de-naturalize it, and replace it with collective stories that open up critical engagements between the expert practitioners and knowledge generators and the embodied experts whose wheelchairs glide smoothly when the road is cleared of debris and rubble. She concludes her article with a semi-imagined composite interrogation:

> "'What did you do to yourself?'
> I have composed myself as a disabled person, a Paralympian, a supercrip.
> 'When did you become disabled?'
> Most recently? Just now.
> 'How did it happen?'
> Through your questions, my answers, these stories, your gaze.
> 'What's your disability anyway?'
> Disability itself.
> 'Are they working on a cure?'
> We are. Are you?"

I am trying to … That is what I have been doing in this book. I haven't tried to reinvent medical sociology, health-care practices or public policy. I've been telling the stories of my *embodied* life at the Bellemont.

On the Writing of
After a Fall: A Sociomedical Sojourn

There are some sixty people who speak in *After a Fall.* They are not composites and they are not characters. They are people. I have tried to honor their humanity. Everyone has some saving grace. Friends and family gave me permission to include them in the text and to quote them. I changed the names and identifiers of staff and residents. And, because there are five rehabilitation facilities seven minutes from my home, the site of the autoethnography is concealed, as well.

Four interlocking *ways of knowing* have driven the writing of this book: sociological, ethnographic, literary, and memory. The writing cuts across disciplinary and cultural landscapes because the ways of knowing intersect, angle off, or travel along together in tandem, creating what I think of it as a *sojourn*, a little journey across time and space.

The working title of this book was *Kisses in the Dark,* to signify that no matter how bleak things may seem, there are little unexpected pleasures to be had. The title has changed but the subtext has not. All writing is an ethical activity. Choices are made. I have tried to write well and truly and to inspire right actions and good spirits in myself and my readers.

What has stayed in my ears these past months are not the alarm bells at the Bellemont, or the "Help me's" or the "moans and grunts" or the West African accents of the nurses. What I hear is the old woman in the long-term wing saying over and over again into the air, "Kiss me... Kiss me." She was not asking for very much—she was not asking to be held, or cured, or brought home, or for changes in the health-care system. She was asking to be recognized, touched gently with another's breath of life, her own breath of life comingling. I hope this book is a kiss.

Acknowledgments

I would be remiss if I did not first acknowledge the support for my work from the qualitative research community. This community has sustained, accepted, and encouraged my intellectual journey. I would also be remiss if I did not acknowledge the support I have had over the decades from the National Science Foundation, National Institute of Education, National Endowment for the Humanities, National Institute of Health-Vocational Administration, National Institute of Health, and The Ford Foundation. These grants and fellowships had allowed me the freedom to pursue my research interests. Some of the findings from different research projects have been enclosed in this book

Special thanks to the people in my book. Orthopedic surgeon Dr. Gregory Berlet. My ankle is stable, my scar near invisible. Thank you! Physical and occupational therapists, nurses and nurses' aides, maintenance and business staff at the Bellemont rehabilitation facility. All of you have contributed to my recovery. Thank you! Fellow Bellemont residents, for telling me your stories, letting me into your lives. Thank you! Dr. Ruane, and physical therapists Scott and Judy at the MacConnell Spine, Sport, and Joint Center who strengthened my ankle and resolve after I came home. Thank you! And, my deepest gratitude to my friends and families who visited, sent cards, emails, gifts, and stuff to eat. Thank you for allowing me to use your *real* names in this book.

My Memoir Writing Group—Bev Davis, Diana Newman, Linda Royalty, Erica Scurr, Linda Thomas, and Deanne Witiak—have been a constant source of wisdom and support, critiquing this book in chunks in drafts, and in its near final form, listening to my worries, engaging in my conversations. Ellyn Geller, Maggie Kast, Susan Knox, and Julie White gave me valuable positive feedback. Repasts with members of my Artist's Way and PMS groups have fed more than my stomach. My friends—Nan Johnson, Patricia Lynch, and Tina Thonnings—have been especially kind and generous during my recovery. My Papillons, Bashi and Lily, have nudged me into taking them for walks—no matter how short the walk, they have continued to love and comfort me.

My editor, Mitch Allen has been, as usual, an ally and a critic. He has pushed me to explicate the implicit sociological dimensions of this book, and I think it is the stronger because of that. The staff at Left Coast Press and designer Detta Penna have created a good looking book.

My husband, Ernest Lockridge, has stood by my side through my surgery and rehabilitation, painted the picture for the book's cover, took on all household tasks and walked, walked, walked the dogs. He has listened to and read every word in this book—more than once, gently coaxing me through the book's sixteen drafts. *Have I said "Thank you"?* Thank you!

The first quoted text appearing on page 262 is from page 59 of Nancy Mairs' 1996 book, *Waist-High in the World: A Life among the Nondisabled*. The second quoted text appearing on page 263 is from Danielle Peers' 2012 article, Interrogating disability: the (de)composition of a recovering Paraolympian. *Qualitative Research in Sport, Exercise and Health* 4 (2), 175-188.

About the Author

Laurel Richardson is Professor Emeritus of Sociology at The Ohio State University. In this book she brings her distinguished career full-circle by revisiting her post-doctoral research interests in the Sociology of Science and Disability Studies. She is an internationally renowned qualitative researcher with specialties in gender, contemporary theory, and arts-based research. She is the author (or co-author) of several hundred articles and seven previous books: *Dynamics of Sex and Gender; Writing Strategies; The New Other Woman* (translated into six languages); *Gender and University Teaching; Travels with Ernest; Last Writes: A Daybook for a Dying Friend;* and *Fields of Play: Constructing an Academic Life,* honored with the Society for the Study of Symbolic Interaction's prestigious Cooley Award. She lives in Worthington, Ohio with her husband, Ernest Lockridge, her Papillon dogs, Bashi and Lily, and her rescued cats, Mimi and Asia. "There is always time for what you do first in the morning," she says. On most mornings, she writes.

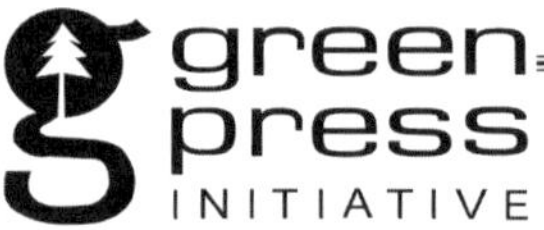

green
press
INITIATIVE